Permanent
and Reconstructive Tattooing

Eleonora Habnit

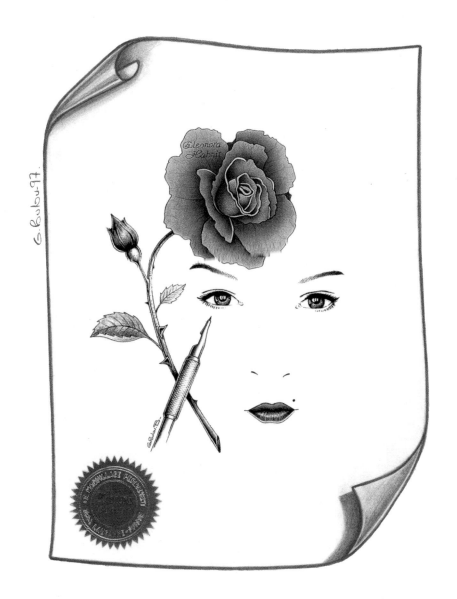

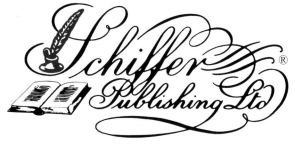

4880 Lower Valley Road, Atglen, PA 19310 USA

Dedication

To my daughter, Emilie.

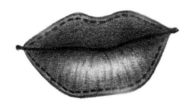

Library of Congress Cataloging-in-Publication Data

Habnit, Eleonora.
　　　(Tout savoir sur le maquillage permanent. English)
　　　Permanent makeup and reconstructive tattooing/by
Eleonora Habnit.
　　　　　p. : cm.
English translation by Anne-Marie Glasheen and Bret Rudnick.
　　　ISBN: 978-0-7643-1833-7 (pbk.)
1. Skin--Surgery. 2. Surgery, Plastic. 3. Permanent makeup. 4.
Tattooing.
　　　[DNLM: 1. Reconstructive Surgical Procedures--methods.
2. Tattooing. 3. Cosmetics. 4. Skin-surgery.
WO 600 H116t 2003] I. Title.
RD520.H3313 2003
617.4'77--dc21
　　　　　　　20030065511

Designed by Ellen J. (Sue) Taltoan
Typeset in Van Dijk/Souvenir Lt BT

ISBN: 978-0-7643-1833-7
Printed in China

Schiffer Books are available at special discounts for bulk purchases for sales promotions or premiums. Special editions, including personalized covers, corporate imprints, and excerpts can be created in large quantities for special needs. For more information contact the publisher:

Published by Schiffer Publishing Ltd.
4880 Lower Valley Road
Atglen, PA 19310
Phone: (610) 593-1777;
Fax: (610) 593-2002
E-mail: Info@schifferbooks.com

For the largest selection of fine reference books on this and related subjects, please visit our web site at **www.schifferbooks.com**

We are always looking for people to write books on new and related subjects. If you have an idea for a book please contact us at the above address.

This book may be purchased from the publisher.
Include $5.00 for shipping.
Please try your bookstore first.
You may write for a free catalog.

In Europe, Schiffer books are distributed by
Bushwood Books
6 Marksbury Ave.
Kew Gardens
Surrey TW9 4JF England
Phone: 44 (0) 20 8392-8585;
Fax: 44 (0) 20 8392-9876
E-mail: info@bushwoodbooks.co.uk
Website: **www.bushwoodbooks.co.uk**

Acknowledgments

My warmest thanks to the illustrator and authors mentioned in the book, to Jeffery Lyle Segal[1] for his sound advice and suggestions, to Marie Brinkley for her invaluable help and enthusiasm, and to those I love who gave me nothing but encouragement.

—Eleonora Habnit
www.thepermanentmakeup.com

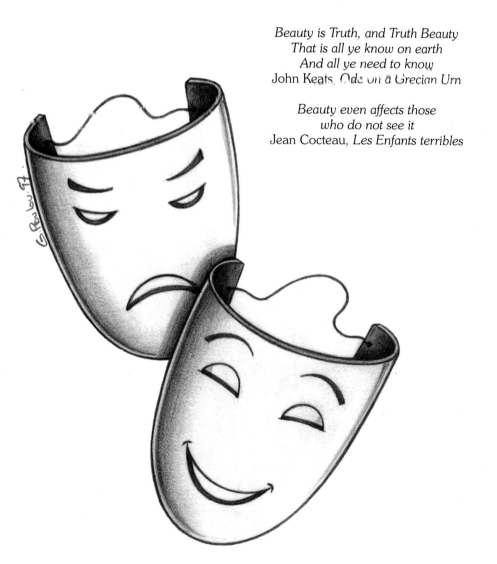

Beauty is Truth, and Truth Beauty
That is all ye know on earth
And all ye need to know
John Keats, *Ode on a Grecian Urn*

Beauty even affects those
who do not see it
Jean Cocteau, *Les Enfants terribles*

Foreword

Micropigmentation or permanent makeup offers the client a means for cosmetic or reconstructive enhancement. There was an important need twenty years ago to disseminate this knowledge to practitioners. Thus, I wrote the first textbook on this subject and a subsequent second edition ten years later. Now with all the new improvement in machines, techniques, colors, and indications, a new book has been written to continue this important flow of information for both the practitioner and consumer.

I applaud the wonderful efforts of Eleonora Habnit and her new book.

In this well written and detailed book, the reader will appreciate all the new developments in micropigmentation since the last textbook some ten years ago. Thanks to her efforts, we now have a new platform of knowledge to share with all practitioners and potential clients.

It is an honour to write this foreword for her book and I wish her much success in the dissemination of this book on an international scale.

—Charles S. Zwerling, MD, FACS, FICS
Founder and Chairman of the American Academy of Micropigmentation
www.micropigmentation.org

Contents

Part 1: Introduction

Chapter 1
Dermagraphics, or Marking of the Skin

"Beauty is only skin deep"
—Chinese Proverb

Every artist has an individual method of expression. An artist uses a "medium" which best suits the need. A painter may choose canvas over wood, a sculptor may choose between stone or clay.

In dermagraphics[1], the "medium" is quite unique, since it is alive and differs from one person to the next. The human skin is a miracle of delicacy and suppleness. It is much more than a canvas; it is a link between the person and the outside world. Like a billboard, it conveys a message to others. Like a photo, a person's skin can bring a variety of emotions to those who look upon it.

The skin, above all else, is a place of exchange. For an artist, working on the skin is no more than an expression of artistic passion. But like the actor, there is the opportunity to quite literally "get into a character's skin" and connect with those who view the art.

Dermagraphics falls into three categories:

✓ Decorative tattoos
✓ Permanent makeup
✓ Reconstructive or paramedical dermagraphics

All three are a type of tattooing, as pigment is introduced into the dermis by means of needles. The pigments are made from the same ingredients, with the exception of ink, which is used mainly in decorative tattoos. The same machines are often used. So, what distinguishes one from another? As we are about to see, the differences lie in their objectives.

Decorative tattoos

Decorative tattoos have probably been around for as long as humanity itself. Originally they were ritualized, incorporating into the self elements from the outside world as a permanent symbol. Perhaps this was a desire for immortality, a way to attract the attention of the gods to help a person survive a hostile world or vanquish an enemy. The most common substances used to dye the skin were black soot collected from cave walls, red earth, and sometimes vegetable matter. Thorns from trees or fish bones were frequently used as needles to carry the pigment into the skin.

Tattooing remained virtually unchanged for thousands of years. In the 21st century, mechanization and modern pigments have made the art of tattooing more accessible than ever before.

Almost anything of a graphical nature is possible when it comes to tattoos, and almost anything goes. People can express the wildest fantasies when it comes to choosing the subject of a tattoo, where it is applied, how large an area to cover, and how colorful it should be. Facial tattoos are usually avoided, but with permanent makeup, it is the face that receives pigmentation.

The majority of those interviewed for a study recently carried out by the Geneva Institut d'Etudes Sociales gave more than one reason for considering a tattoo, which is why the total number of replies exceeds 100% (see table below).

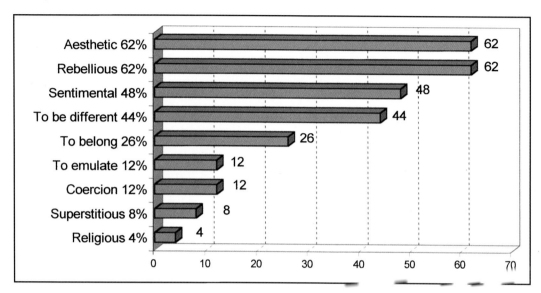

Reasons that would lead interviewees to consider getting a tattoo.
From a study carried out recently by the Geneva Institut d'Etudes Sociales[2].

Permanent makeup

A beautiful face is an advantage greater than any letter of recommendation.
—Aristotle

Permanent makeup is a relatively recent phenomenon, becoming more prevalent in the last fifteen years. It is not an extreme art but one of subtle harmony. Tattooing is an alternative to cosmetic pencils applied to the eyebrows, eyelids, lips, cheeks, and other parts of the face.

Decorative tattoos aside, there are two reasons why people go in for permanent makeup: aesthetic and practical.

The words "makeup" and "mask" are related. Both words refer to something that is applied to the face — a kind of "screen" between the made-up person and whoever is looking at that person. Permanent makeup is different in that the pigment becomes one with the body. This can make an enormous difference to a woman because once her makeup becomes a permanent part of her it becomes part of her inner self. Someone who has had permanent makeup will attract attention but the observer will not immediately be able to determine why.

Reconstructive or paramedical dermagraphics

Reconstructive dermagraphics attempts to correct birth defects (e.g., cleft palate), correct disfigurement from illness or accident, or provide cosmetic corrections from some surgery (such as reconstruction of breast areolas, scar therapy, achromia, vitiligo, and alopecia). This is a type of medical intervention.

You might have heard the term "bio-tattoo." It has become fashionable to add the prefix "bio" (from the Greek, *bios*, meaning "life") to give the impression that something is natural and healthy. It is usually a meaningless marketing ploy. There are people who think that "bio-tattoos" are not long-lasting, or that "more natural" pigments are used. However, there is no such thing as a "bio-tattoo." It is a tattoo.

When it comes to permanent makeup, there are those professionals who are uncomfortable referring to the word "tattoo" because of the stigma that lies behind it. But, in all honesty, permanent makeup is a form of tattooing.

These days all three areas of dermagraphics have benefited from a more scientific approach. Science has discovered much regarding the stability of pigments and the skin's ability to tolerate them. It has aided in creating a greater number of regulations governing hygiene and sterilization. It has assisted in communicating experiences on a professional level in papers and conferences. It has studied the equipment used in application, and much more. It forms a bridge between "decorative art" and medical art, and is, in this respect, invaluable and irreplaceable.

Whether ancient (decorative tattoos), more recent (permanent makeup), or medical (reconstructive applications), dermagraphics has always sprung from the same deep-seated desire of man, or rather woman, to be pleasing to oneself and others. It is no coincidence that "to please" comes from the same root as "pleasure": it is a pleasure to please. Dermagraphics therefore clearly contributes to pleasure, and therefore to happiness.

You're under my skin
There's nothing to be done
You're everywhere
On my body
I'm cold...
I'm hot...
My skin I feel
Is feverish
—Gilbert Bécaud/Jacques Pills,
Sung by Edith Piaf

[1]From the Greek *derma*, "skin," and *graphein*, "to write."

[2] Ivo Fibioli, Cosette Gigandet, Gabrielle Pugin, *Tattoo-Tabou. Etude d'un phénomène social: le tatouage et les réactions qu'il suscite*, (Tattoo-Taboo, Study of a social phenomenon: tattoos and reactions to tattoos), Geneva, p. 31.

Chapter II
Permanent Makeup:
An Affair of the Heart

But I, Narcissus, am simply interested
In my own essence:
To me all else has but a mysterious heart,
Oh my very sovereign dear body, I have nought but you!
The most beautiful of mortals can only cherish himself...
—Paul Valéry,
Fragments of Narcissus, Charms

Biologically speaking man would
be unable to weather the stresses of life
if he did not have a few pleasures in which to indulge.
—Henri Laborit, *l'Homme et la ville*

In dermagraphics, every step must be planned with care, beginning the moment a client steps across the threshold. At my Institute, for example, flowers and music create an atmosphere that helps women relax and puts them at ease.

From the moment she walks through the door, each and every client becomes the most important person in the world to me. I listen to her, treat her with respect, and get her to give me an account of her life so that I can build up an image of how she sees herself. We are usually quick to strike up a conversation that is both frank and open. She then fills out a questionnaire regarding her medical background. What I glean from her responses forms the basis of our discussion.

The work unfolds on several levels: psychological, technical, and artistic. In other words, one deciphers the real reason behind the consultation. It is important to be realistic so that one can determine what is technically feasible. It is also important to establish a proven track record when it comes to the harmony of shapes and colors.

There are occasions when women want the impossible. Perhaps they have been misinformed. The most difficult situation I am faced with is when a woman is chasing a dream or wants to recapture her lost youth. She is in a way expecting something that I cannot give her.

"When it comes to applying makeup to the bruises of the soul and the ills of the body, the gesture becomes an act almost identical to therapy. Cancer is one of the ills that makeup cannot cure although it can contribute to alleviating the effects of the illness. For a woman to lose her hair, eyebrows and eyelashes as a result of chemotherapy is a dreadful trauma which only exacerbates the illness."[1] Eyebrows and eyeliner can be tattooed. "This changes how they see themselves and how others see them too. [...] From a therapeutic point of view, to make oneself up is to bring into play the same relational codes we have with our surroundings. This is something that can be found in all cultures."

A beautician stated that "during the recent Bosnian war, I was surprised by what the woman requested: we were sending them the basic necessities of life and they were asking for lipsticks. They claimed it stopped them from going crazy, that it helped them cling to reality. In certain circumstances, makeup can become a basic necessity."

However, the majority of women simply want to look more attractive.

Permanent makeup has the added advantage of being timesaving and practical. These days, time is a precious commodity. Twenty minutes saved each day represents a saving of one hundred and twenty hours a year! Permanent makeup can give you back a week or more in a year, not to mention all that time spent on the chore of removing makeup.

Although one cannot put a price on beauty, the initial investment in permanent makeup can soon be recovered. Consider the time saved by no longer having to apply and remove conventional makeup, and also the savings made by not having to buy cosmetics and makeup removing products.

We are no longer and should never again be slaves to femininity. The women of today can, at the same time, have a profession, be in love, be mothers, be sportswomen, and a whole lot more. In this way they can have meaningful private and social lives. They want to have it all, and why not, but with a minimum of effort and without being overly burdened every day in the process.

Thirty years ago, a social revolution saw women burning their bras. Shrewd and determined, women retrieved them along with their makeup bags, and today with permanent makeup. The outstanding success of the latter is admittedly no more than a token, but a substantial one for all.

"Everything falls into the logic of individual arbitration, what I would call self-government and which is the very logic of modern individualism. The principle of free self-determination has touched the feminine...Recent studies have shown that the more a woman works, the more she takes care of herself. Her appearance no longer comes second. A working woman goes to the hairdresser more often than a housewife does. She uses more makeup. She keeps an eye on her figure and is more sympathetic than others to cosmetic surgery. She "works at" her appearance. Her personal contribution to the work is not made to the detriment of her wish to look good and to seduce...It is the taking responsibility for one's own destiny. It is the modern rejection of fate."[2]

[1]Isabelle Cerboneschi, "Makeup to counteract the ills of the body and the bruises of the soul," from the *Nouveau Quotidien*, 21 August 1997. All quotations in this chapter come from this article.

[2]Gilles Lipovetsky, interview from the *Nouvel Observateur*, 30 October to 5 November 1997, discussing his book *La Troisième Femme*, Gallimard, 1997.

Chapter III

Who Benefits and What Can Be Done?

Who benefits?

✓ Men and women of all ages
✓ Anyone interested in saving time
✓ Women who want twenty-four hour a day beauty and comfort
✓ Women who hate makeup that streaks or rubs off
✓ Sports enthusiasts of all kinds
✓ People with poor eyesight who wear contact lenses or glasses
✓ Women who are allergic to conventional makeup
✓ People wishing to correct certain facial asymmetries
✓ Accident and burn victims and people with disfiguring scars following surgery
✓ People suffering from loss of pigmentation
✓ People suffering from alopecia (loss of body hair), whether permanent or temporary (e.g. following chemotherapy)
✓ Women with shaky hands or the physically handicapped
✓ Women who want to restore "unfortunate" dermapigmentation.

In other words, a lot of people!

What can be done?

Eyebrows

• Too light or fair
• Broken by a scar
• Partial alopecia
• Badly positioned or asymmetrical
• Eyebrows too low or drooping
• Patchy or swirling eyebrows
• Insufficient eyebrows — too short
• Lack of eyebrows
• Surgically damaged or scarred

Eyeliner and kohl-line

• For a deeper more seductive look
• When eyelashes are too fair
• When eyelashes are scant or lacking
• For women whose eyes are inclined to water in the wind, cold, light, etc.
• For people with poor eyesight

Lips (outline and full lips)

- Because lip pencil and lipstick rub off when eating, smoking, and kissing
- Lips too thin
- Lips asymmetrical
- Lips too thick
- Badly or undefined outline
- Lips too pale
- Scars resulting from an accident
- Cleft-lip disfigurement

Beauty spots and freckles

- Just for fun
- To disguise minor imperfections or scars (e.g., chickenpox, acne)

Blusher

- For the sheer pleasure of looking healthy...

Areolas of the breasts

- To camouflage scars following surgery for reduction or enlargement
- To recreate areolas, to give the illusion of nipples
- To darken pale areolas
- To enlarge small areolas
- To redefine irregular outlines

Camouflaging scars or depigmentation

- When you are fed up with seeing them (and showing them...)

Alopecia (hair loss)

- To create the illusion of hairs or hair

To summarize

A growing number of women no longer want to spend time putting on makeup. They want to be as beautiful in the evening as they are in the morning, not to mention at night!

In short, whatever your lifestyle, permanent makeup is for you. No one will even notice you have not made yourself up as usual.

Who should you contact?

Making the decision is the easy part. Now comes the difficult part: finding the right person to make your dream come true. It is particularly important to make the right choice, therefore it is imperative that you spend as much time on this as you would in choosing a doctor or dentist. After all, you will be placing your face, your appearance, your personality in this person's hands. He or she must be a fully qualified professional.

First, we suggest you visit any establishment under consideration in order to check that there is a room reserved exclusively for the application of permanent makeup (to ensure no bacteria from other activities will be found, e.g. hairspray, nail dust, etc.). It must be spotlessly clean. There should be sterilizers in view and rubber gloves should be worn while the work is being carried out. The chair should be covered in protective paper. The needles should be in sterile wrappers. In short, everything must exude perfect hygiene and inspire confidence.

You should also check the technician's professional qualifications. Find out how long they have been practicing. Did they go to a special school? If so, for how long? Have they upgraded their skills over the years? (This is an area in which technology is evolving rapidly.) Inquire about the number of treatments they have done.

If you are contemplating permanent lipstick, scar camouflage, blusher, or another specialist treatment, insist that the technician has the necessary qualifications for this type of work, since it is far more specialized than permanent makeup on the eyes, eyebrows, or lipliner.

Another crucial factor concerns your file and any follow-up. Will the establishment keep a special file on you? Have they asked you to fill in a questionnaire on your general health? Are they willing to guarantee long term follow-up, particularly with regard to "touching up" when this becomes necessary? Do they ensure confidentiality?

To sum up: *Always think long term.* Permanent makeup is a tattoo that you will be wearing for a long time. You should "feel good" or "have a good feeling" about the person who will be applying it so that you can establish a relationship based on trust. The success of your permanent makeup depends on this.

Chapter IV

How Is It Done?

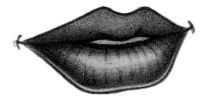

How is it done?

Permanent makeup is the introduction of specialized pigments, specially produced for dermapigmentation, into the dermis, or deeper layer of skin, by means of one or more needles.

Does it hurt?

Thanks to the wide availability of local anesthetics (I use these automatically), in theory the procedure is no more painful than having your eyebrows tweezed.

Who decides on shape and color?

More often than not, the client is in control here. They usually know what they want and what best suits their face and personality. Most technicians try to respect the client's wishes as long as these are within the bounds of what is considered aesthetic. (Each client is, after all, a walking testimonial for some time to come.) Quite often, however, clients do ask for advice or put themselves entirely in the hands of their technician.

Do you first do a drawing?

Yes. It is essential to first sketch the "project" with a cosmetic pencil in order to appreciate what the final effect will be, and to experiment until the client really "feels" it is right. The drawings are all executed with the person standing or sitting, as features change when you lie down.

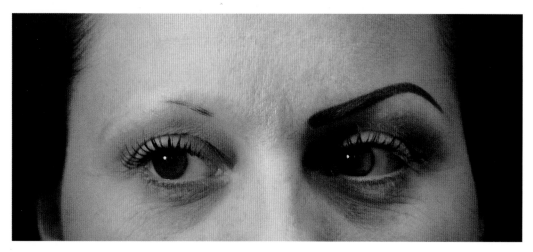

Drawing the eyebrows prior to cosmetic tattooing.

How do you select the color?

The goal in color selection is to match the desired shade of pencil or makeup. In order to determine a match, liquid pigment is dabbed onto the skin, close to the area to be pigmented (on the forehead for the eyebrows, for example) so that the effect will be as life-like as possible.

Will I be presentable on the actual day I have permanent makeup?

For between four to six hours, the area treated will be slightly reddened and swollen. However, due to water retention, the eyelids can remain puffy for twenty-four to forty-eight hours in around fifty percent of cases. The effect is similar to how you might look if you had been crying. By the following day, application and removal of your everyday cosmetics is allowed. However, for around four to six days, the pigmentation will appear somewhat obvious, dark, and intense. By day seven, the epidermis (or top layer) flakes and peels, sloughing off the remaining pigment, to leave the color softer.

Is permanent makeup really permanent?

How long it lasts will vary enormously depending on a variety of factors. These are:

- The color selected (each color has a different life expectancy)
- How much time the individual spends in the sun (the more time you spend in the sun or tanning bed, the faster the color fades)
- The speed of cellular regeneration (the longer it takes cells to regenerate, the longer the color lasts)
- The phagocytosic capacity, in other words, the "absorption" of the pigment by the organism
- Depth of implantation of pigment (approximately one to two millimeters depending on the area)

Permanent makeup fades more rapidly on the face than on the body as it is permanently exposed to daylight. Ideally, the color should be touched-up every two or three years depending on how well the pigment holds. With some people, makeup fades after a year while with others there is no change after eight years.

The word "permanent" is used because the molecules that make up the pigment remain in the skin for life even when they have grown very faint[1]. It should be noted that in Latin, *permanere* does not signify "lasting forever," but rather "lasting for a long time."

Is there any risk of infection or contamination?

No, as long as:

- The needles are sterile and used only once
- The facility is clean
- The technician is wearing gloves
- The skin is disinfected prior to treatment
- An antibiotic cream is used following the procedure

How much does it cost?

Prices vary considerably. How the quality relates to the price is far more important than the price itself. A factor to be taken into consideration is whether the cost of permanent makeup includes the price of touching up.

At present, the average price for treatment ranges from $400-500 in salons and from $500-800 in physicians' offices. Prices are also subject to regional variations.

Will it look natural?

In theory, permanent makeup is designed for daytime wear. To add a touch of glamour for the evening, add a little pencil. How many of us would want to take our children to school dressed as though we were going to a nightclub? Moderation is recommended at all times. It's like seasoning your food: once it's there you can't take it out. But if, after a month, the permanent makeup is really too light, it can always be intensified. And it is a widely held belief that permanent makeup – well-applied –looks more natural than pencil makeup.

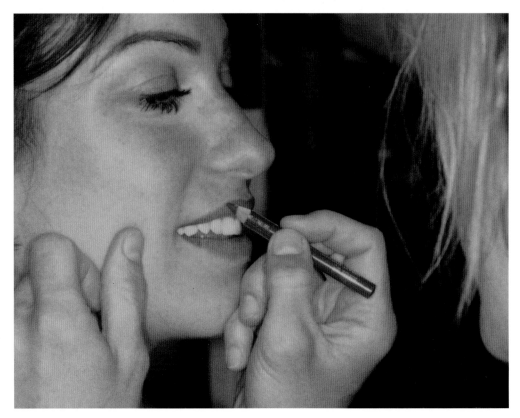

Drawing the lipliner.

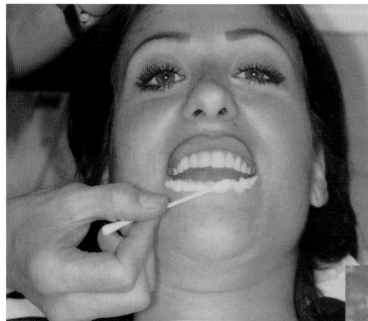

Applying local anesthetic.

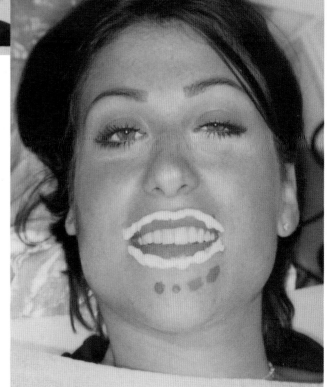

Selection of color.

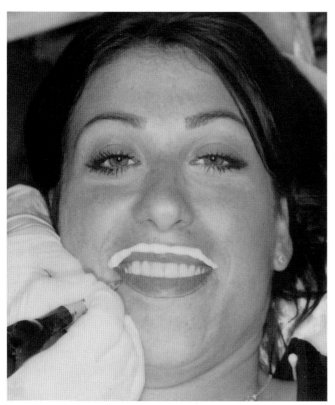

Tattooing the lower lipliner.

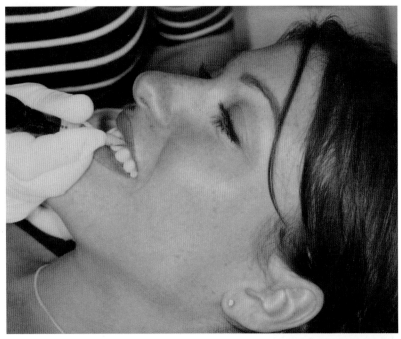

Tattooing the upper lipliner.

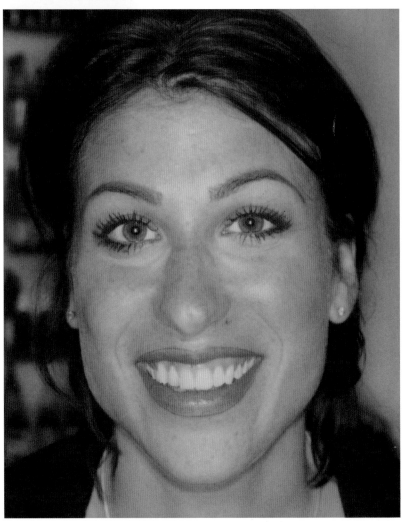

The final result immediately after the procedure.

[1]A woman went to court in the United States because she claimed that her permanent makeup had disappeared and that she had therefore been misled by the term "permanent." However, she lost the case as the judge ruled that the makeup was indeed permanent because there were molecules remaining in the skin. *Permanent Press*, Society of Permanent Cosmetic Professionals, July/August 1997, p. 11.

Chapter V

And After?

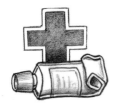

After care: On the first day, it is advisable to apply antibiotic cream or ointment until the client goes to bed.

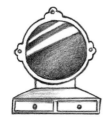

Cosmetics: On the second day, makeup may be applied and gently removed. Rubbing must be avoided.

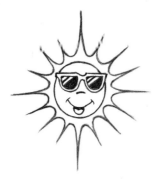

Sun and tanning beds: No direct exposure *for ten days*. If this is not possible, protect the pigmented area (wear a hat and sunglasses) and apply a "total sun block" cream.

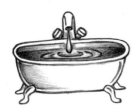

Water: Avoid *prolonged* contact with water (shower, bath, swimming pool and sauna) *for four to six days*. Regarding the lips, brush teeth and rinse after meals, in order to remove all traces of salt and acidity. Afterwards, apply lip balm if necessary.

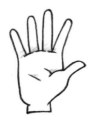

Itchiness: This is a sign that the treatment is healing. On no account should the flakes of skin and tiny scabs that form be scratched or picked, as this will remove the color. The flakes fall off around day six.

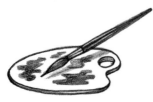

Color: The pigmentation will appear very obvious, dark, and intense for four to six days. The skin will then flake or peel and the color will look lighter and softer. It will lighten still further before stabilizing after a month.

Dermapigmentation is not so much a science as an art and the reaction of each and every one of us will be different.

Chapter VI
Equipment

Every trade has its tools, and this profession is no exception.

It is not the intent of this chapter to grade, according to quality, the different tools used for permanent makeup. What is important is that the user feels comfortable with the implement, and that it is a pleasure to use. A violin is not "better" than a flute; a piano is not "superior" to a double bass. The chosen instrument depends on the musician's taste, training, and artistic awareness, and above all what kind of "couple" he and his instrument make. In much the same way that permanent makeup becomes part of the skin, so the implement, with experience, becomes part of the person using it, as though the hand had been biologically extended.

Whatever the shape, name, or origin, the equipment used in dermagraphics can be divided into three categories depending on how they operate:

✓ Manual tools (ancient implements consisted of splintered bone, sharpened bamboo sticks, etc.)
✓ Reciprocating coil machines
✓ Rotary pens

People sometimes speak of the superiority of a particular "electronic" machine over manual tools. As a term, "electronic" sounds very modern, but it is not altogether correct. There is nothing electronic about the dermagraphic machine itself except the speed regulator.

Moreover, we can straightaway dismiss a frequently expressed fear: whether the electric machine rotates or vibrates, the electricity is never in contact with the skin. All it does is drive the motor. One is no more likely to get an electric shock during the tattooing process or the application of permanent makeup than from dialing a telephone.

Manual tools

Manual technicians can claim their techniques have been around the longest since they go back to the dawn of time. Electric tools have only existed for a little more than a hundred years.

Anywhere from 1 to 150 needles are attached to the end of a holder. In the past, this was made of wood or bamboo. These days, it is usually made of plastic or metal. The technician dips the needles into the pigment just as he would a pen. He then introduces the pigment by pricking the skin. To increase the intensity of color, the skin must be struck several times in the same spot.

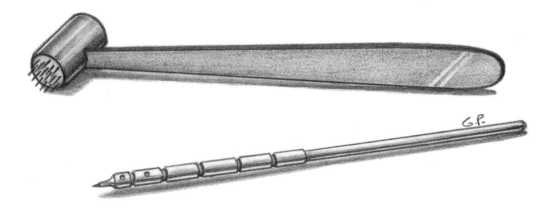

Unlike electrical machines, where the needle moves inside a tube that is a mini-reservoir containing pigment, manual implements have no reservoir and they must therefore be repeatedly dipped into the pigment. With this method it does take much longer to produce the desired result. Since "patience is a virtue," under the circumstances the term "patient" is most appropriate. This method does, nevertheless, produce some exquisite tattoos and permanent makeup.

What are its advantages and disadvantages? The implement, which is of course silent, is extremely light and consequently easy to handle. It is also cheap since there are no mechanical components. But, as mentioned earlier, it does require a great deal of patience.

When it comes to the application of blusher[1], a small round mallet fitted with several spaced-out needles is sometimes used. This mallet — which looks a little like a toothbrush — has a flexible handle, thus allowing the operator to pat the skin more systematically in order to introduce the pigment.

Reciprocating coil machines

It was in 1880 that the American Samuel O'Reilly first invented the tattoo machine, although it was his English cousin Tom Riley who patented and exploited it in 1891.

Here the needle is connected to a metal rod that alternately strikes the end of one or two magnetic coils about 75 times a second. It is based on the same principle as that of an old telephone bell (one of the old telephone bells, rather than a modern electric one). If you listen carefully to one of those bells, you will hear that the sound is not actually continuous. The blade rapidly and repeatedly strikes one or two small metal "bells." The blade is activated by one or more magnetic bobbins that first attract it, and then, when the current is cut for a few thousandths of a second, release it, then attract it once more and so forth. This machine can look slightly amateurish, for the needle is held in place with a rubber band. (However, it should be remembered that rubber bands are used in many areas, even in high-tech machines and medicine.)

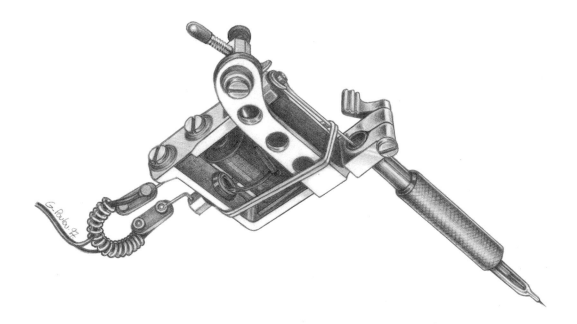

What are the advantages and disadvantages? Although these machines are not particularly attractive to look at, they have a certain "retro" charm: all the components are visible. They are heavier to handle, but they are more powerful than rotary pens, an indispensable quality — in the case of reconstructive applications — when harder or thicker skin (e.g., scar tissue resulting from burns or surgery) has to be penetrated.

The machines do not run on batteries but are powered by direct current, through a fairly large transformer[2] and/or power supply. While they are much noisier, they are solid and sturdy. And since the components are exposed to the air, they cool more quickly and can therefore run all day long. Moreover, thanks to ease of access, it is not difficult to maintain and replace components.

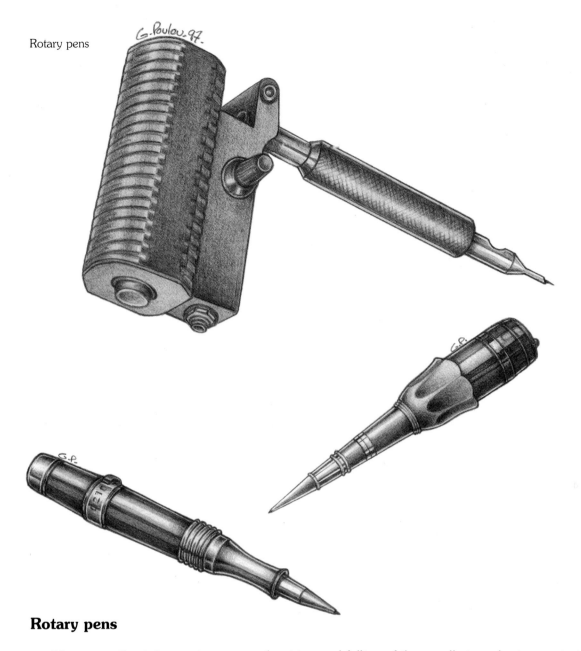

Rotary pens

Here a small rotating motor powers the rising and falling of the needle in order to penetrate the skin. For some time now, man has been capable of transforming alternating movement into rotating movement and vice versa: e.g., the piston engine in a car transforms the *alternating* movement of the (rising and falling) pistons into the *rotating* movement of the wheels. In an electric sewing machine, the opposite takes place: these machines are driven by a *rotating* motor, and this rotating movement is then transformed into an *alternating* movement so that the needle can rise and fall. Basically the rotary pen is much like a mini-sewing machine.

What are the advantages and disadvantages of rotary pens? They are more attractive. The pens are light and pleasing to handle. Since they require very little current, they can run on batteries, transformers, and/or power supply. They are also relatively quiet.

The newest type of these machines is the "digitally" controlled, cosmetic tattoo machine. Its technologically advanced digital control unit (power supply) assures a more consistent needle speed and depth of the penetration.

In conclusion, and in response to those of you who ask whether one machine is more effective than another, it is less the machine/tool that is *effective*, but more so the artist using it. The key factor is that technician and client hit it off from the start!

[1]See Chapter XIX on "Rouge/Blusher"
[2]The transformer converts alternating current from the national grid into direct current.

Chapter VII
Pigments

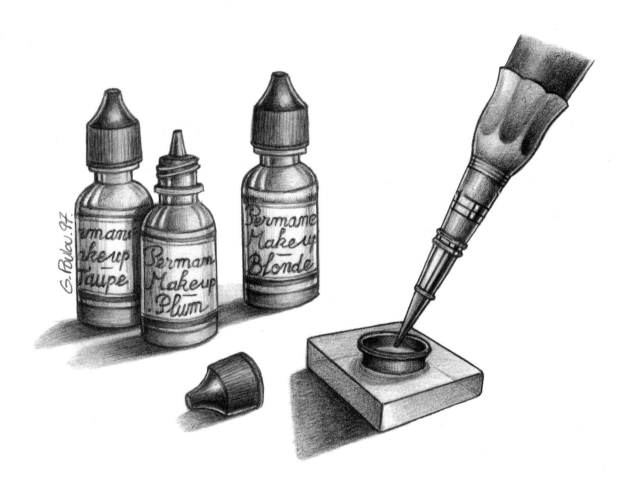

A frequently asked question is, "Are the pigments used in permanent makeup 'natural'?" What people really want to know is whether they are "safe," because they believe that anything "natural" must be "safe."

However things are never that simple. The fungus *agaric* (a red toadstool with white spots) and *hemlock* (the plant that killed Socrates) are deadly poisons even though they occur "naturally." Just because something is "natural" does not necessarily mean the body can tolerate it.

Moreover, the pigment used in tattooing is not a simple dye like food coloring, which passes through the body in a matter of hours. (Fortunately we do not turn green whenever we eat pistachio-flavored ice cream.) The quest for a "natural" substance with which to pigment the skin will not necessarily lead to a substance that is swallowed.

Furthermore, the cosmetic industry these days no longer uses natural pigments; they are all synthetic. Nowadays the pigments used in permanent makeup are:

✓ Organic
✓ Inorganic

Organic pigments

Organic pigments used to be made from living organisms, vegetable or animal, and are essentially carbon derivatives. Carbon is the base of organic chemistry. This is no longer the case today: for the most part they are products of synthesis born of carbon chemistry. They are a combination of organic and carbon materials. Why carbon? Because this element combines so perfectly with itself as well as with other elements that they can never be separated. In other words, these pigments are virtually indestructible.

The three most frequently used elements in the synthesis of these pigments are hydrogen, oxygen, and nitrogen. They are to be found everywhere and, depending on the quantity and position of the substances combined with carbon, allow the great number of tonalities desired.

These organic pigments disperse in the skin. This means that, as the main constituent of the human body is water, they will dissolve over a period of time. To prevent the color from dissolving, the soluble organic pigment is combined with an insoluble substance, such as hydroxide of alumina, which "coats" the pigment[1]. The coat is relatively heavy due to the fact that it contains a metallic element. The pigment becomes heavier and as a consequence acts as a fixative, which holds better under the skin. The coat also renders the pigment molecule insoluble in the human body. Lastly, the added advantage of this procedure is that it reduces the risk of an allergic reaction because the "coat" isolates the organic substance in the body.

Contrary to what might initially be thought, experience has shown that organic pigments, whilst they are admittedly brighter, are much more likely to cause an allergic reaction than iron oxide, which is the basis for the majority of inorganic pigments.

The lighter colors are generally composed of organic pigments whose life expectancy is shorter than that of inorganic pigments. Consequently, permanent makeup based on organic pigments runs the risk of fading more rapidly than when it is based on inorganic pigments.

Inorganic pigments

Inorganic pigments are derived from ores. One of the most commonly used — in the manufacture of black, brown, flesh, etc. — is iron oxide. It is also the best tolerated. But not all colors can be obtained from this substance and other metals have to be used.

As well as the organic/inorganic duality, there is also the natural/synthetic duality. Through the process of synthesis, we can now create substances that are as organic as they are inorganic. Synthetic perfume is already commonplace; molecules with the scent of one flower or another are artificially produced in a laboratory. Inorganic substances are likewise synthetically produced, especially as the extraction of certain ores is forbidden, presumably to protect some of these deposits from running out[2].

To sum up, inorganic pigments or minerals are primarily used in dermagraphics. These are more often than not produced synthetically from metals. Iron oxide is the most widely used.

It is quite understandable that clients should be curious as to the *composition* of inorganic pigments. However they should also know about their *structure* and *properties*. Ideally, the pigments used in dermapigmentation should reveal the following characteristics: absence of toxicity, stability when subjected to light, insensitivity to metabolism, and absolute insolubility. The particles are monitored so that their size is in the region of six microns[3] or more. This is to ensure that their stability remains constant and that they do not spread.

Pigments come in powder form. To be used in dermapigmentation, they have to be in a liquid form. In order to achieve this, they are suspended in an antiseptic solution, usually made up of alcohol, glycerin, and/or distilled water.

A few examples to illustrate the composition of cosmetic pigments

White This color has a titanium dioxide[4], zinc oxide, or barium sulfate base
Yellow Derived principally from yellow arylide
Red Either red selenite or alizarin
Blue The most common organic blue is made from a phtalocyanine base and ultramarine from aluminosilicate of sodium
Green Produced from chrome oxide or phtalocyanine
Violet Magnesium oxide base
Brown Ferrous oxide Fe_2O_3
Black Ferric oxide Fe_3O_4 or carbon

This chapter might read like a chemistry lesson, but those who prefer diagrams to text may find the following tables on the manufacture of pigments easier to understand. Don't let them dissuade you from adding a little pigment to your life!

[1]Anglo-Saxon literature uses the term *lake* ("lac"), as though the particle were "lacquered."

[2]The German company Beyer and the American company Dow Chemicals are two of the world's biggest suppliers of iron oxide. However, an infinitesimal amount of their output goes into tattooing.

[3]And not three microns, as in the black of ink.

[4]It has been found that titanium dioxide-based white can help prevent cold sores, by acting as a sunscreen.

PIGMENT MANUFACTURING

POWDERED PIGMENT

(Fine, Insoluble Powder, Solid Particles)

MIXED (SPECIFIC FORMULA)

(Isopropyl Alcohol, Glycerin, Water)

MILLED

(Measure: i.e. Particle Size Control & Uniform Size)

Using a specific technique that consistently reproduces the pigment product with certain specifications :

SHADE

VISCOSITY

CONCENTRATION

PARTICLE SIZE

Specific formula (blend of colors)

To create other shades, for example for a color chart

ORGANIC COMPOUNDS
(Anything Relating To Life)

Carbon based

Carbon

Element that combines with itself and other elements (Chains Pure Carbon = Diamond, Graphite, Coal)

There are over a hundred elements. The three main elements able to combine with carbon to form pigments are

- Hydrogen
- Oxygen
- Nitrogen

These combinations of elements are molecules

The properties of these molecules are that they can absorb and radiate different wavelengths that correspond to a specific color.

In terms of cosmetics, it can be derived from natural ingredients such as plants, animals vegetables

D&C Dyes are synthetic made carbon products certified by the FDA for topical cosmetic use

IRON OXIDE
(SYNTHETIC)

Iron + Oxygen + Sulfur = Iron Sulfate

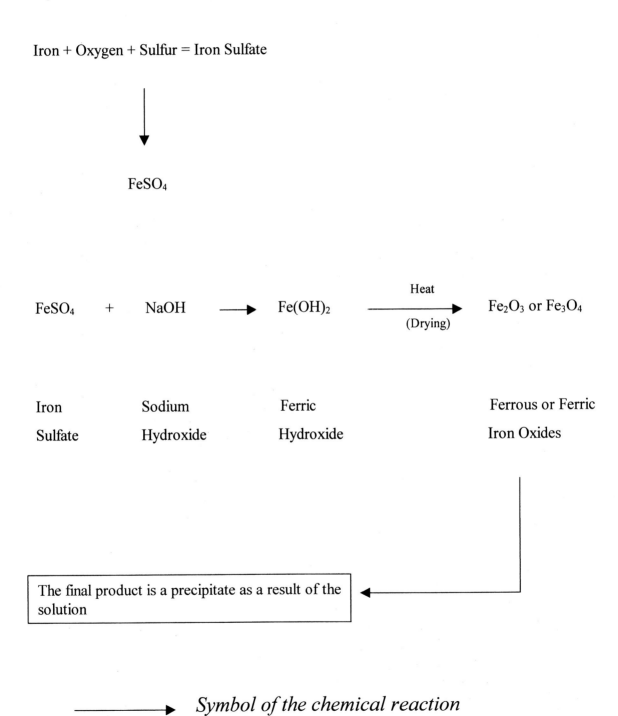

$FeSO_4$

| | | | Heat | |
| $FeSO_4$ | + | $NaOH$ | $\longrightarrow$ | $Fe(OH)_2$ | $\xrightarrow{\text{(Drying)}}$ | Fe_2O_3 or Fe_3O_4 |

| Iron | Sodium | Ferric | | Ferrous or Ferric |
| Sulfate | Hydroxide | Hydroxide | | Iron Oxides |

The final product is a precipitate as a result of the solution

$\longrightarrow$ *Symbol of the chemical reaction*

IRON OXIDE
(NATURAL)

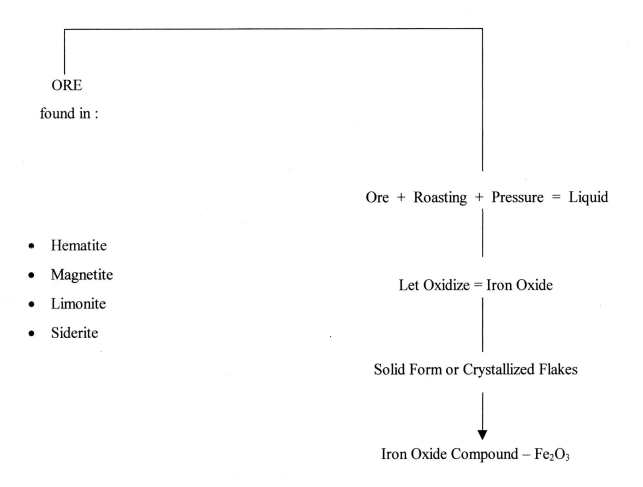

ORE

found in :

- Hematite
- Magnetite
- Limonite
- Siderite

Ore + Roasting + Pressure = Liquid

Let Oxidize = Iron Oxide

Solid Form or Crystallized Flakes

Iron Oxide Compound – Fe_2O_3

The quantity of oxygen and how long heat is applied determines the color.

The heat gives different forms of iron.

Physical form gives color.

All four charts courtesy of Darlene Story, www.lipigments.com, © Lasting Impression I, Inc.

Chapter VIII
Color Theory

*In reality, we work with very few colors.
What gives the illusion that there are many,
is that they have been put in their rightful place.*
—Pablo Picasso[1]

Since the dawn of time man has been fascinated by the colors of the rainbow. And yet, colors do not exist. They are different wavelengths of light. Every object absorbs a part of the waves composed of white light, and emits another that we perceive as a color. Your lips are not red: they absorb all the colors except for the color red, which is sent back to us.

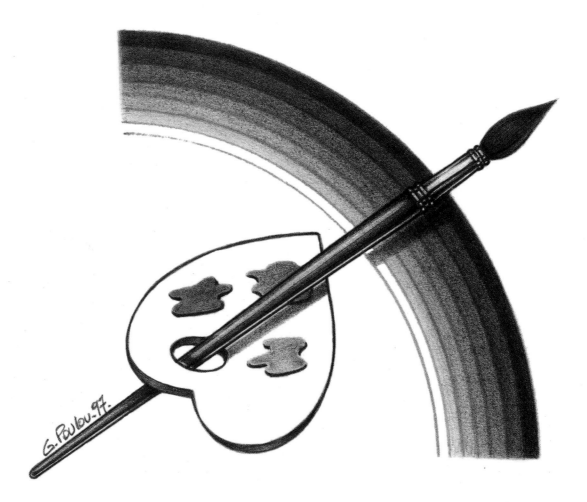

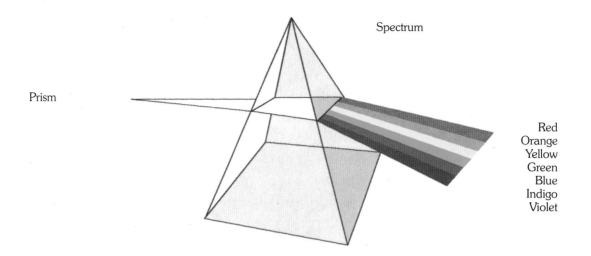

Spectrum

Prism

Red
Orange
Yellow
Green
Blue
Indigo
Violet

The English physicist Isaac Newton (1642-1727) studied color by passing light through a small glass pyramid (prism), thereby artificially recreating a rainbow. He identified the seven primary colors: red, orange, yellow, green, blue, indigo and violet.

It was at the beginning of this century that an artist from Bern, Switzerland, named Johannes Itten (1888-1967) developed the present day theory of color, with his chromatic[2] circle of twelve colors.

Contrary to what many artists believe, the theory of color has nothing to do with having a "trained eye." Like science and mathematics, it is based on absolute rules.

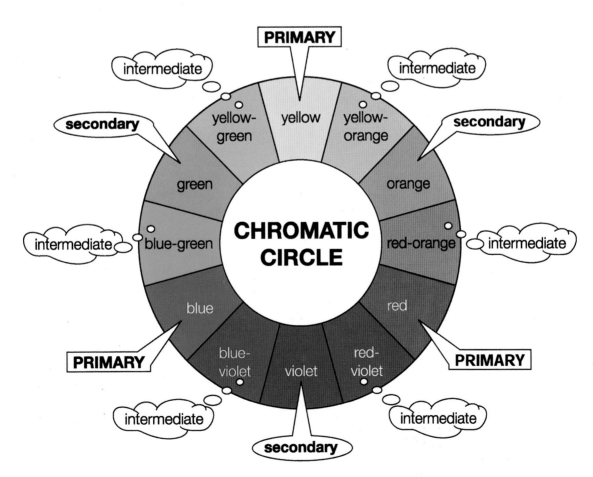

31

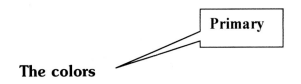

The colors

Blue – red – yellow: these are the *three* basic colors on which all the others are based. They are called "primary" because they cannot be made from other colors.

Blue   The "strongest" of the primary colors. It adds coolness and depth.

Red   With medium "strength," it adds warmth and fullness.

Yellow   It is the least "strong," the clearest, and the brightest of the colors, the only one that can add warmth and coolness.

Because the primary colors have different strengths, you need:

* Twice as much yellow to obtain the same strength as red
* Three times as much yellow to obtain the same strength as blue
* Twice as much red to obtain the same strength as blue

Relative strength of colors: 3 x yellow = 2 x red = 1 x blue

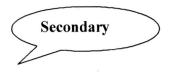

Colors

According to the formula of relative strengths above, two primary colors must be combined to create the three secondary colors.

Orange   2 parts red + 3 parts yellow

Green   3 parts yellow + 1 part blue

Violet   2 parts red + 1 part blue

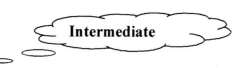

Colors

An equal parts mixture of one (single) primary color with one (single) neighboring secondary color creates the *six intermediate colors:*

Yellow-*orange*	(3 parts yellow) + (*2 parts red + 3 parts yellow*) = **3 parts yellow + 1 part red**
Red-*orange*	(2 parts red) + (*2 parts red + 3 parts yellow*) = **4 parts red + 3 parts yellow**
Red-*violet*	(2 parts red) + (*2 parts red + 1 part blue*) = **4 parts red + 1 part blue**
Blue-*violet*	(1 part blue) + (*2 parts red + 1 part blue*) = **1 part red + 1 part blue**
Blue-*green*	(1 part blue) + (*3 parts yellow + 1 part blue*) = **3 parts yellow + 2 parts blue**
Yellow-*green*	(3 parts yellow) + (*3 parts yellow + 1 part blue*) = **6 parts yellow + 1 part blue**

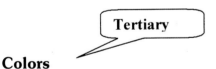

Tertiary

Colors

All the other color combinations, a few examples of which are listed below:

✓ Ochre	✓ Taupe	✓ Plum
✓ Blonde	✓ Fawn	✓ Cherry
✓ Amber	✓ Indian earth	✓ Fuchsia
✓ Khaki	✓ Rust	✓ Mauve
✓ Buff	✓ Wine	✓ Lilac
✓ Bistre	✓ Bordeaux	✓ Jade
✓ Brown	✓ Garnet	✓ Olive
✓ Tobacco	✓ Ruby	✓ Turquoise
✓ Havana	✓ Purple	✓ Moss

Most of the colors used in permanent makeup are tertiary colors.

Transparent and opaque colors

Contrary to what is generally believed, the colors used in permanent makeup and for tattoos are for the most part transparent. Afterwards, they get progressively darker as more is added. In color theory this is known as *volume*.

The majority of colors have volume. Hence the application of several layers of a red tonality will make blusher darker and deeper. Therefore, if you apply a second layer of the same tonality, the result will be darker.

This is best illustrated by way of an example:

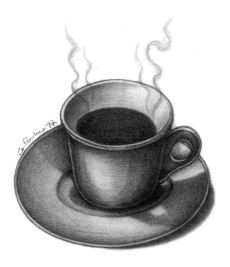

Let us compare the color of coffee when you look at it in a cup and when you look at it in a spoon: the color is the same but the *eye* does not perceive it as being so. The coffee appears to be light brown in the spoon but virtually black in the cup.

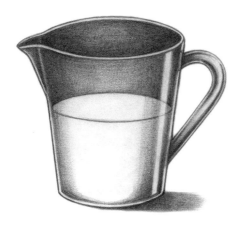

However, white is not a color that has volume. Volume has no meaning in this case. When you look at milk, whether it is in a jug or a spoon, it looks the same. The smallest drop of white has the same intensity and the same density as a greater volume.

In permanent makeup and in tattooing, some colors are chosen for their *transparency* and others for their *opacity* and their ability to mask or camouflage.

Don't "fall" for just any color though! The colors that attract us don't necessarily suit us. There is a natural harmony between the skin tone and the color of the hair and eyes. The wrong choice of color in permanent makeup can upset this balance and give the disturbing impression that "something is not quite right." On the other hand if you "play your cards right" a color could be your trump card!

When all is said and done, and theory aside, color can have a considerable psychological, emotional and aesthetic impact. To play with colors is to create emotions in oneself and others. As Johannes Itten said: "their intrinsic essence is hidden from our intellect, only intuition is capable of understanding it"[3].

[1]Conversations with Christian Zervos, *Cahiers d'Art*, 1935.
[2]From the Greek *chroma*, "color."
[3]*Art de la couleur,* abridged and revised edition, Dessain and Tolra, Paris, 1966, p. 94.

Chapter IX

Why and How to Identify Skin Tone

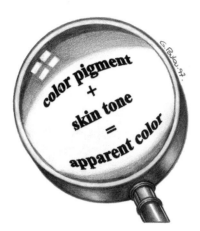

Unlike applying makeup to the skin with a cosmetic pencil, permanent makeup is introduced into the skin, or more precisely, into the dermis. Every skin has its own tone, which acts as a color filter that modifies the apparent color of the implanted pigment. These skin tones are identifiable and appear in the "color wheel" below. So as to avoid any unpleasant surprises, it is absolutely vital to determine your skin type and its base tone.

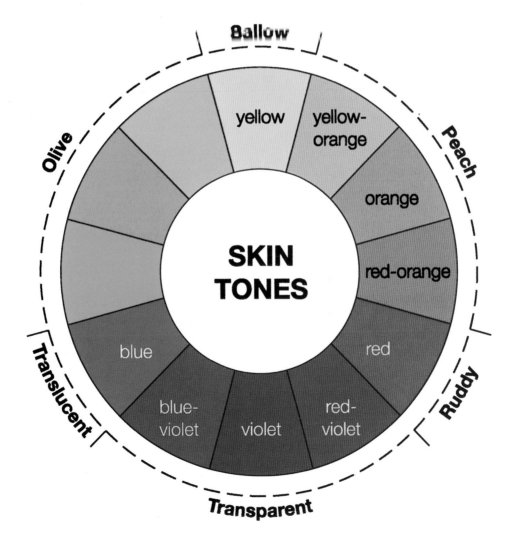

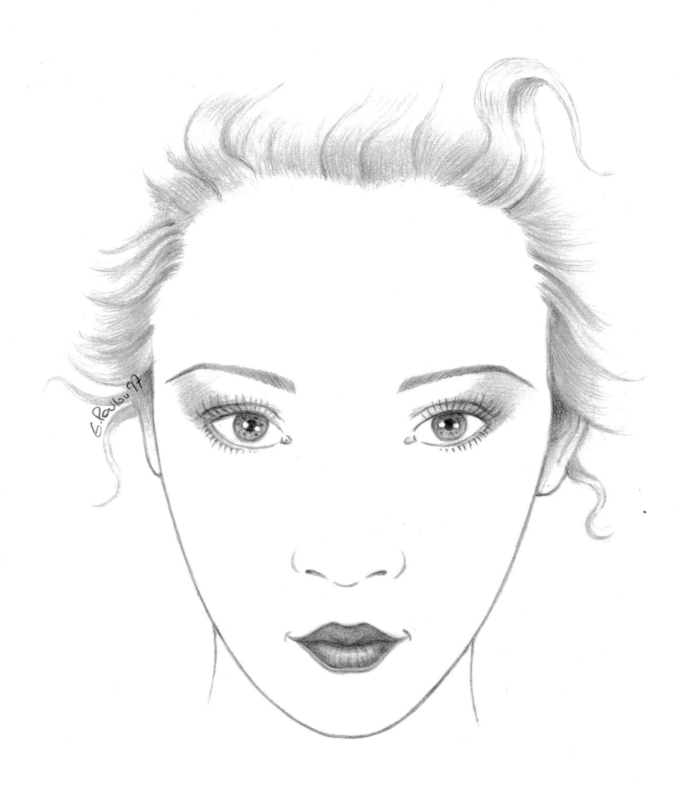

36

Transparent[1]

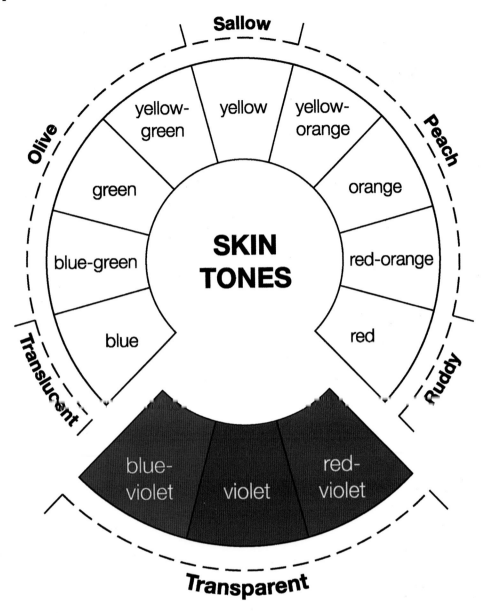

Red-violet, violet, blue-violet.

These are skins with irregular skin tone. The skin is often delicate, the area surrounding eyes and lips often reddish-violet or reddish-blue. Typical of transparent skins is a yellowy-orange or red mottled effect.

These are skins with fair ascendancy, including pale Anglo-Saxon or Scandinavian cool alabaster to pale beige. Hair may have been platinum or ash blonde in childhood and turned to a darker shade of ash brown as an adult. Ash greenish-brown color or grayish-brown undertones are present.

This client is a prime candidate for altering her hair color. She may streak her hair or add more red or gold highlights (sometimes fighting with their natural coloring). Check for hair color grow-out or eyebrow color, unless this too has been changed. Clients feel and look pale without cheek color.

Around the eyes and lips, veins may show, leaving a reddish-violet or bluish-violet tinge of color.

The base tone of this skin is

red-violet, violet or blue-violet

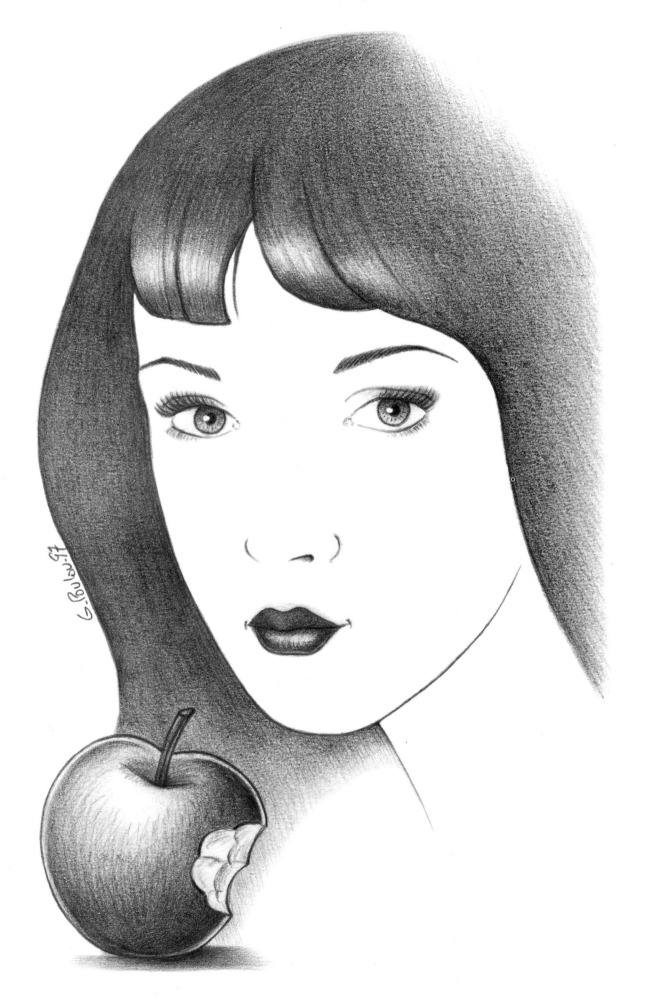

38

Translucent[1]

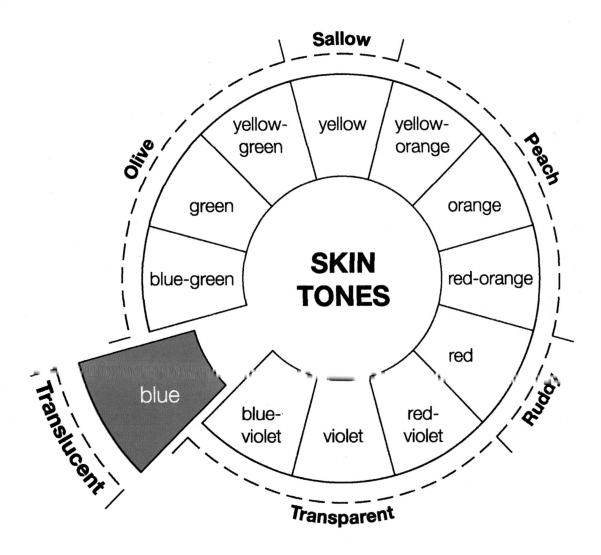

Blue, extremely white, or extremely black, no median value.

There is an element of density in this complexion.

There is a clear blue milky undertone to the skin. The client may be like Snow White with dark hair and pale skin. The hair may be dark brown or near black, making a sharp contrast to the milky whiteness of the skin. There is no pink cast.

This client tends to gray early in life and usually colors her hair from the time she is in her early to mid-thirties.

The base tone of this skin is

> *blue*

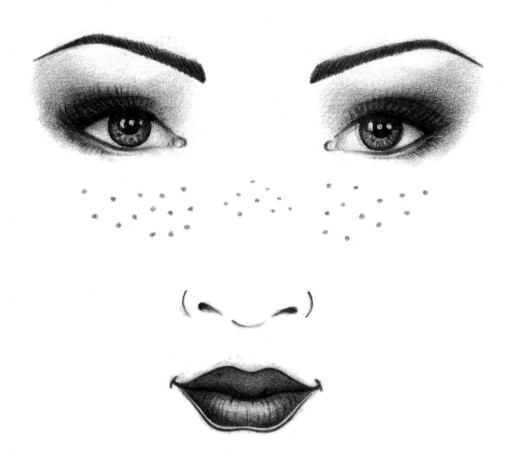

Ruddy complexion[1]

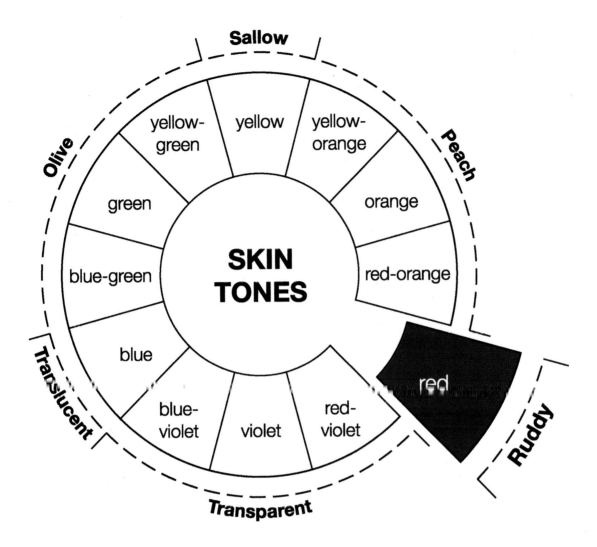

Pink, coral pink with tinges of color.

This complexion will have obvious red undertones.

This client will have a rosy red or ruddy cast to the skin. It may range from a delicate shell pink to a much deeper tone. Ears will have a tendency to be pink. Eye color will be brown or green, occasionally turquoise or aqua. Hair color ranges from golden blonde, strawberry blonde, to reddish brown or rich copper shades.

Frequently these clients will be freckled. As they age, more ruddiness and freckling becomes apparent. The hair color will tend to be a yellow-gray.

The base tone of this skin is

> *red*

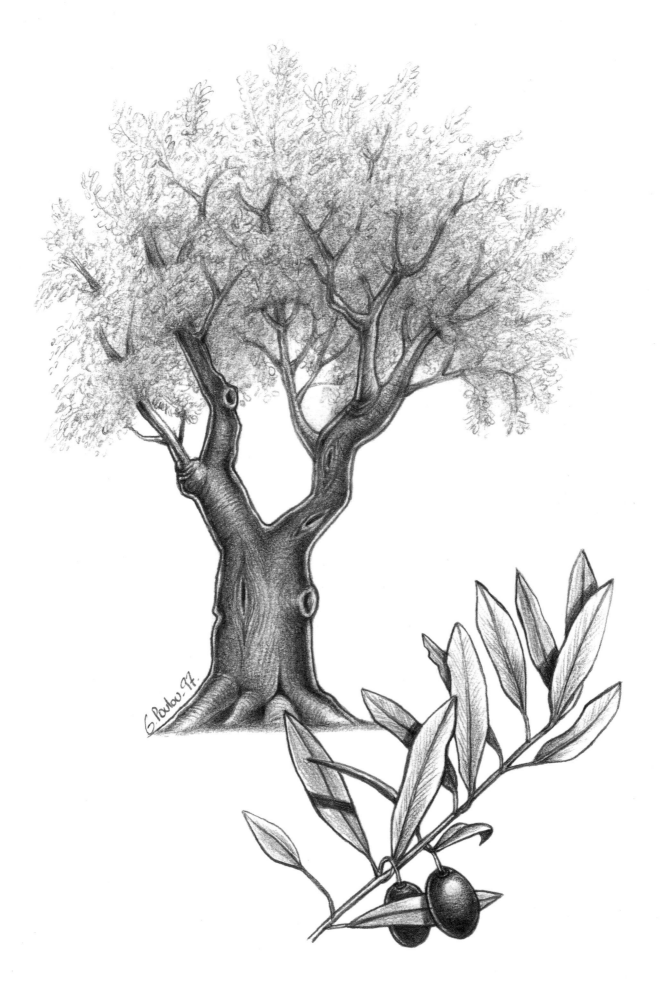

Mediterranean, olive[1]

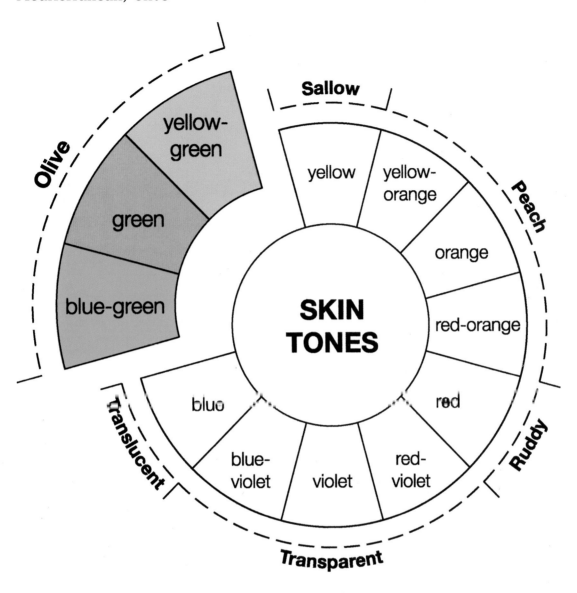

Yellow-green, blue-green, or combination skin.

Pale-olive (yellowy-green) complexions are often difficult to assess.

Olive skins with a cool green or bluish-green cast to the skin. They are true brunettes with very dark eyes. People from Spain, Italy, and other coastal Mediterranean countries share these characteristics. Their skin is devoid of natural red tones. The Hispanic woman may have a paler skin color, but the same undertones. The cheek color has a strong, clear, slightly blue-red undertone.

The base tone of this skin is

green or blue-green

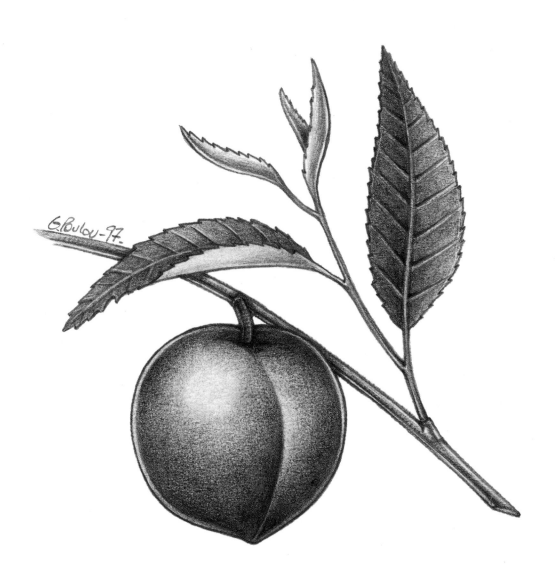

44

Golden girls, peach[1]

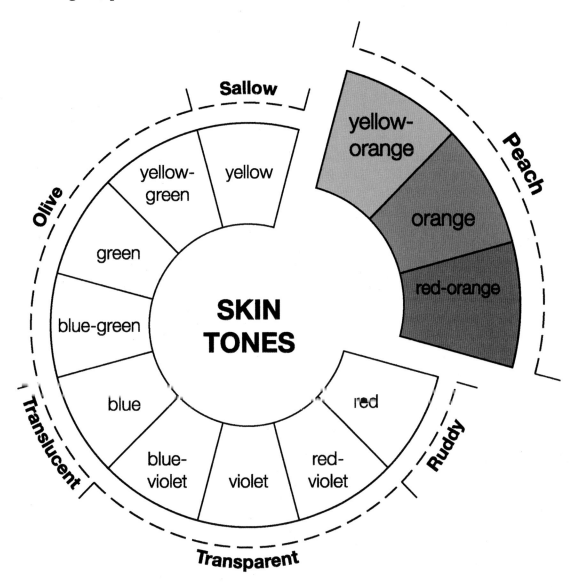

Yellow-orange, orange, red-orange. A peach tone can have red tints. This "peachy" complexion is *never uniform.*

Also known as peaches and cream, this skin range from pale honey or ivory to the richer bamboo tones. The fairer of these clients will have peaches and cream complexions and blush easily. Their hair tends to be ash blonde, flaxen, or golden blonde but may be a richer, deeper golden brown or strawberry blonde.

They do not blush as easily as those with ruddy or rosy complexions. Their hair will pick up a yellow cast as it grays.

The base tone of this skin is

yellow-orange

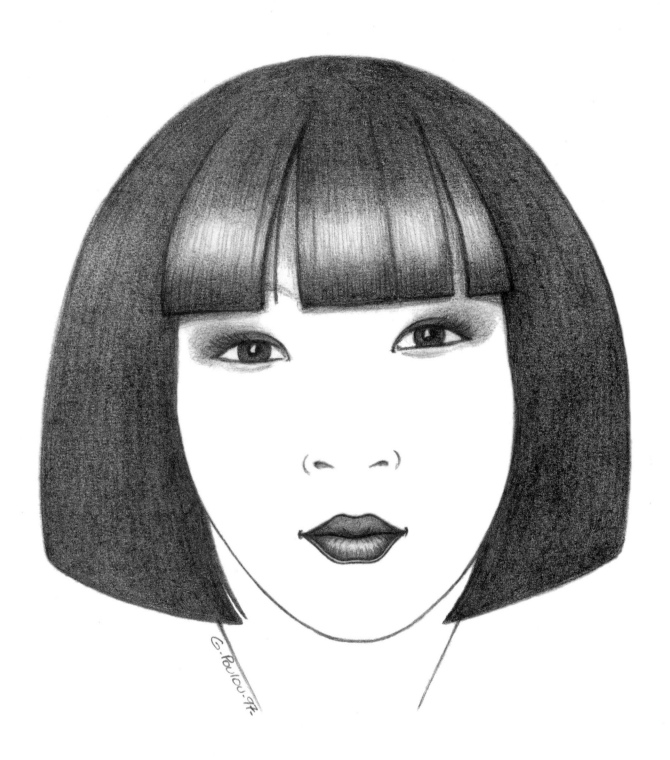

Asian, sallow[1]

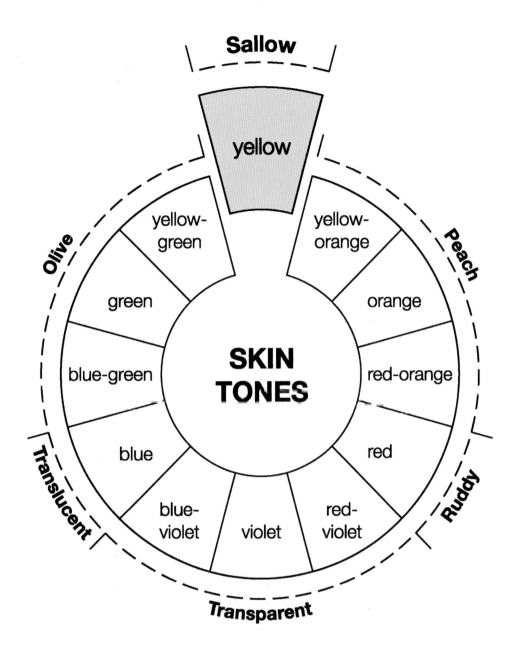

Yellowish, warm or cool, can take on yellow-orange or yellow-green tones.
This skin tans.

Sallow skin tones with pale yellow-based or ivory skins without the greenish or olive tinge of the Mediterranean. If there is any greenish tinge present, it is a yellowish-green with no blue cast. Their eyes and hair are dark with no red or coral undertones to the skin.

The base tone of this skin is

yellow or yellow-green

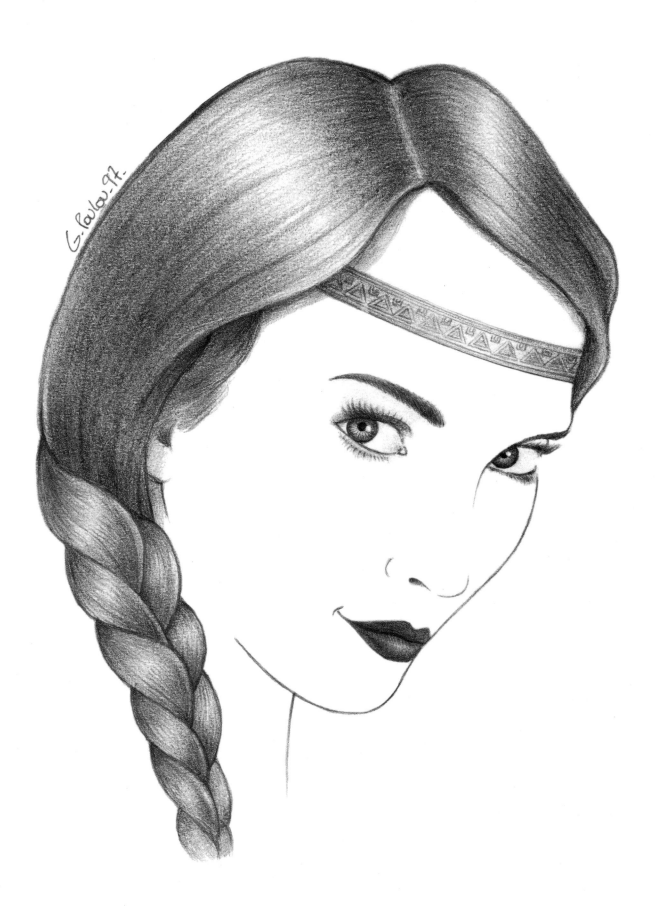

48

Native American Indian, peach[1]

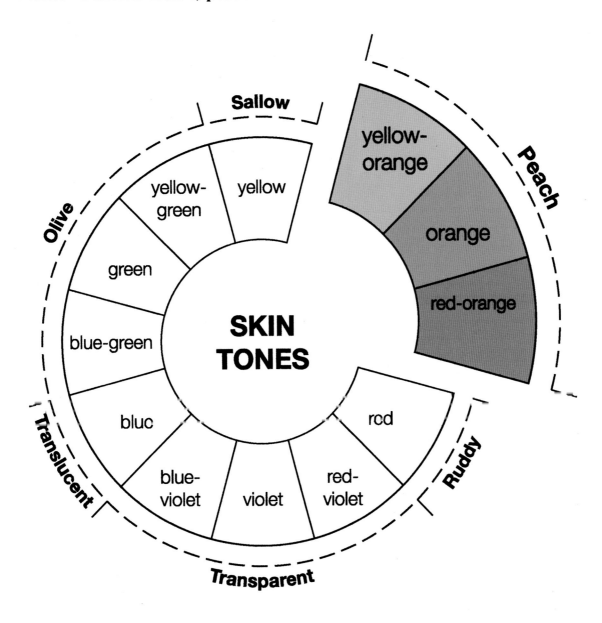

Yellow-orange, orange, red-orange.

A peach tone can have red tints. This "peachy" complexion is never uniform.

These clients are often mistaken for Mediterraneans but they generally have a warm skin undertone. Their skin is actually in the peaches and cream category with an "orangey" red cast. Some Hispanic skins fall into this category, as their ancestry may actually be a blend of Native American Indian and Mediterranean.

Think warm bronze or copper, rich and deep tones that accent their dark, near black hair and eyes.

The base tone of this skin is

> **_orange or red_**

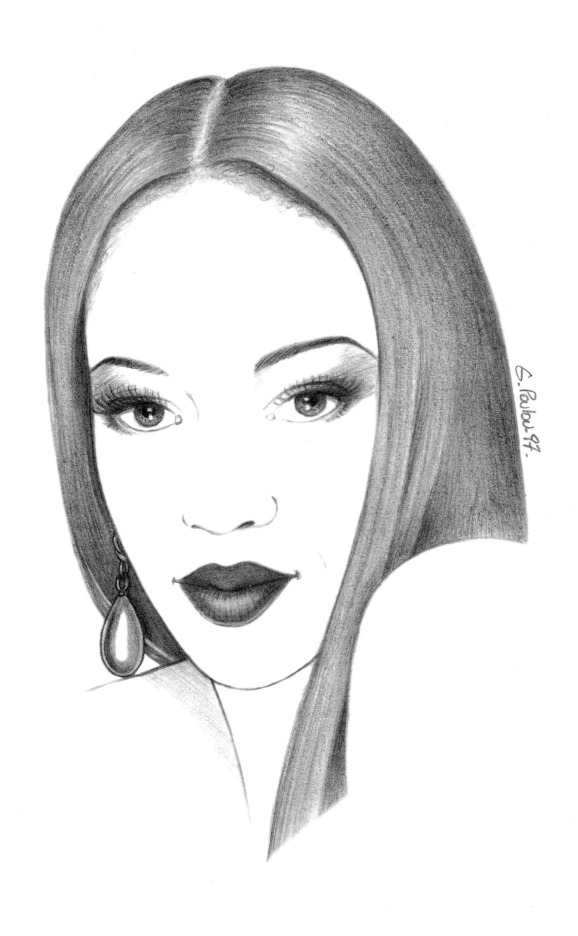

50

Women of African Descent[1]

These clients most commonly fit into the Mediterranean (olive), translucent (blue), or American Indian (bronze) skin tone categories. Use the above guidelines to determine which best suits the individual.

Each skin-tone group can also be classified according to its quality and saturation point. Dark skins are not always olive or translucent and pale skins are not always transparent or sallow.

In making determinations, do not be fooled by the presence of red tones that are a result of sun damage and the aging process. Other factors can come into play.

All skin thins with age and therefore tends to show the veins under the skin more often. Additionally, all skins will tan within their own color range and each color category can have skin tones ranging from fair to deep. But it is also true that the deeper a person's tan the more red and yellow tones appear. All hair will bleach with sun exposure, picking up red and gold tones.

Amongst the other factors likely to affect skin color and its underlying tone, we should mention that there are certain illnesses and medicines that will do this, as will tanning pills!

[1]Information © Culp Ent. Inc. With the courtesy of Judith Culp, who has developed a skin tone kit, available at *www.permanentcosmeticsnw.com*, which will allow skin type and underlying tone to be easily identified within a matter of minutes.

Chapter X
Light and Color

Ex luce ars
Ex arte lux

From light comes art
From art comes light

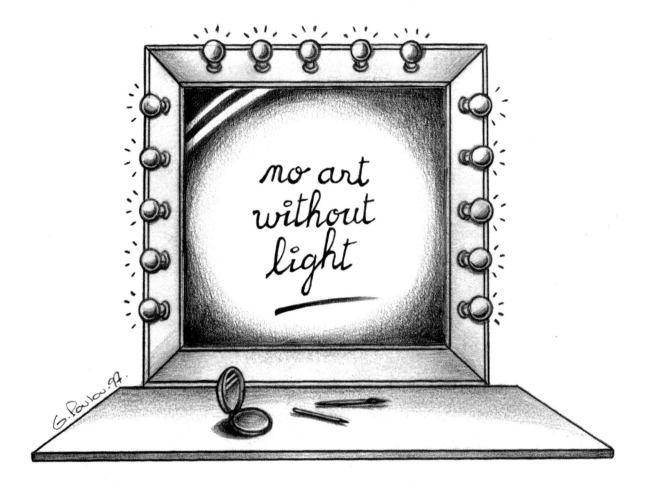

Color would not exist without the following three elements:

- An object
- An eye
- An illuminant

Take one away and color no longer exists. It is really important to understand that color is a physical sensation, a perception.

Colors can look different depending on the lighting. We have all had the experience when shopping for clothes — the color is no longer the same outside in broad daylight as when you get home.

It is an undeniable fact that colors are at their best in natural daylight. Around midday on a fine day, the temperature of light is approximately *5,500 degrees Kelvin*.

Even if you are lucky enough to be working near a window, the light is rarely strong enough, especially in winter or when the weather is bad.

So that the "right" color is chosen and to ensure that technicians do not strain their eyes it is essential that certain criteria as regards lighting be respected.

A client, initially delighted with the color of her lipliner, will get a nasty shock later if she looks at her lips in neon lighting and finds that they look like a dark smear of blueberry juice. The light was obviously "bad," in other words too "warm," when her permanent makeup was applied.

In light of this, let us examine the question more closely.

Incandescent light bulbs

These traditional light bulbs (light temperature: around 2,700 degrees Kelvin) make colors look yellow and "warmer" than they actually are. In this kind of lighting, we can be led to believe we see a warm pink color, whereas in effect the pink is made up of cool blue tones that cannot be seen.

Moreover, the older these light bulbs get, the more yellow the light becomes, resulting in a further distortion of color. What should we say then about actors' dressing rooms, with their mirrors surrounded by those small bulbs? It is probably the worst kind of lighting in which to put makeup on!

Halogen lighting

Brighter and whiter[1] (around 2,900 to 3,000 degrees Kelvin) than traditional bulbs, they are a better form of lighting. Moreover, they rarely change color with age. However, their light is still much too "warm."

Fluorescent lighting

From around 3,000 (yellowish light) to around 4,500 (greenish light) degrees Kelvin, fluorescent lighting contains no red tonalities, which makes the lip color deeper and bluer. This does at least have the advantage of preventing too deep or too cool (containing too much blue) a color pigment from being chosen. And, like halogen lighting, fluorescent strips do not change color with age so their light remains constant. Whilst they might not be the ideal solution, they are superior to incandescent or halogen lights.

Artificial daylight lamps

As we have said, colors are at their best in natural daylight. The ideal lighting system is therefore artificial daylight that has the same color temperature, i.e. around 5,500 degrees Kelvin (equivalent to daylight at noon on a fine day).

These special lightings (some are a combination of special fluorescent tubes and incandescent light bulbs) are available in two styles: ceiling lightings or the more common adjustable secondary lightings.

As a client, you are not very likely to be totaling up the number of degrees Kelvin! But if the "harsh" and merciless light of this professional lighting fills you with trepidation, then cheer yourself up with the warm and flattering glow of candlelight.

---

[1]When they are set at maximum power. However, rheostats (dimmers) often control halogen lighting, which means that when the light is turned down it becomes yellow.

Chapter XI

Hyperpigmentation

Hyperpigmentation is an excess of brown pigment in the skin, which some individuals are prone to due to some kind of "trauma." This phenomenon can completely alter the color of permanent makeup, making it a deeper brown or gray-blue tone. It is therefore vital to know which skin types are predisposed to hyperpigmentation.

Some "traumas" are internal in origin. Acne or hormonal changes (e.g. stretch marks or dark patches on the face during pregnancy) can bring them on. Others are external, such as exposure to the sun, the use of tanning beds, injuries, abrasions to the skin, laser treatment, and tattoos.

As the majority of clients do not know if they are prone to hyperpigmentation, it is necessary to search the body for scars or blemishes. These should be carefully examined to see whether, within the scar itself or the immediate surrounding area, there is an area darker than the natural skin — this could be indicative of a tendency to hyperpigmentation. However, not finding any such areas does not necessarily mean the client is in the clear. A predisposition to hyperpigmentation might not show up in one area of the body but it could in another.

In order to gain a better understanding of the possibility of hyperpigmentation, skin type can be divided into six categories according to how it reacts to the sun. This is extremely useful when it comes to ascertaining the likelihood of hyperpigmentation. Our skin color, referred to as the *constituent* color, is governed by heredity. It is the color of the skin found in areas of the body not usually exposed to the sun. We each react differently to sun. It is a tan that will give the skin its *facultative* color.

Skin Type	Unexposed Color	Tanning Reaction*
1	White	sunburn, no tan
2	White	sunburn, tanning difficult
3	White	red, then slow tan (pale brown)
4	Pale brown	red, then tans easily (mid-brown)
5	Mid-brown	seldom red, tans well (dark brown)
6	Dark brown/black	never red, deep tan (near black)

* End of winter reaction (skin as yet unexposed to sun), after 45 to 60 minutes exposure

In the above table, Types 3 to 6 are prone to hyperpigmentation as a result of the different skin traumas described above.

Each of these traumas induces an increase in the amount of melanin the pigment cells (melanocytes) produced in the epidermis. Paradoxically, this overproduction in the epidermis of melanin will occasionally see a corresponding reduction of melanin in the dermis, where it is destroyed by the action of the macrophage cells (melanophages). This turns the skin dark brown (superficial epidermal or dermal melanin) or a more marked gray-blue (deep dermal melanin). This is called post-inflammatory hyperpigmentation (PIH). It usually disappears after a few weeks or months, along with the inflammation, but it sometimes lasts for the rest of one's life.

The human skin is made up of four chromophores (color bearers):

- Melanin (which looks brown or blue depending on how much is in the skin)
- Carotene (yellow)
- Oxygenated hemoglobin (red)
- Deoxygenated hemoglobin (blue)

It is the proportion of these four components that determines the skin's tonality. The *blood flow* would appear to be responsible for "measuring out" blue and red, while brown is determined by *skin type* and *exposure to the sun* and yellow by *diet*.

Ideally, a person prone to post-inflammatory hyperpigmentation should wait weeks, even months, for it to fade. Is there anything that can be done to avoid or cut down this waiting period?

High factor sun lotions used to protect the skin against damage caused by A and B ultraviolet rays inhibit the radiation-induced production of melanin by the melanocytes. These sun lotions can also be used in dermapigmentation.

The same applies to quinol and kojic acid (fungal in origin and weaker) found in "bleaching creams." These products can reduce melanocytic activity. It should however be pointed out that unlike kojic acid, quinol can, if used over a long period of time, *increase* hyperpigmentation — a phenomenon called exogenous ochronosis. Above a concentration of 4% these products are only available with a prescription.

For people who have a history of hyperpigmentation, it would be advisable to begin with a sunscreen lotion followed by quinol or kojic acid prior to tattooing. Application should be repeated about three weeks later, once everything has healed.

A technician who comes across this predisposition to hyperpigmentation — for example, when a client asks that an area of white scar tissue whose edge is darker than the skin color be re-pigmented — might be advised to refuse. There is always a risk that the procedure might provoke the re-emergence of the phenomenon, thereby aggravating the first hyperpigmentation. The client should be informed of this possibility. That said, the majority of cases of hyperpigmentation caused by a micro-trauma like tattooing or permanent makeup will disappear by themselves within three to six months.

When hyperpigmentation exists, the client can ask her doctor to remove the extra melanin through a chemical peeling or short laser bursts. The chemical agents used, either glycolic acid or Jessner's solution, remove the hyperpigmented layers by speeding up the natural exfoliation of these layers. But it is important to bear in mind that chemical peelings and laser treatments are a form of "trauma" that can, paradoxically, (re) induce hyperpigmentation.

When it comes to the skin, whatever its complexion, we must strive for homogeneity. Alas, nature provides us with some unfair competition, for even nature is prone to allowing traumas (sun, scars, etc.) to spontaneously pigment certain areas of the skin! It is up to us to foil these plans.

Chapter XII

The Use of Anesthetics

There are tattoo parlors where I have seen a notice that says: "Yes, it hurts!" It has always been accepted that people with tattoos were tough and that, as with an initiation ceremony, they had to suffer to "warrant" this splendid body adornment.

Is it really true, as the maxim says, that you have to "suffer to be beautiful?" Not necessarily. There are two good reasons why permanent makeup should not be painful:

✓ It is not just for "tough men" but for everyone
✓ It is usually applied to the face, a particularly sensitive area of the body

Should we not, therefore, do all we can (and so much can be done these days) to ensure that any pain will be kept to an absolute minimum or avoided altogether?

When it comes to permanent makeup/tattoos, there are five ways of reducing or eliminating pain, depending on time and place.

Cold

We know that sensitivity to pain is alleviated when the skin is numbed with cold. While permanent makeup is being applied however, the numbness does not usually last long enough for the work to be undertaken. Nevertheless the cold can — depending on the nature of the intervention — provide much appreciated assistance. The most effective method is to use small watertight sachets (first placed in the freezer) that contain a cold-retaining blue fluid, or, failing that, an ice cube (in a plastic bag to prevent the water from running as it thaws). The blue sachets (or ice cubes) can also be used after the treatment, to soothe or relieve swelling.

Mild local anesthetic

The quality and type of anesthetic required will very much depend on the person's age, tolerance to pain, general condition, and state of mind on the day of treatment. Younger and more highly-strung individuals often have a lower pain-threshold.

A wide range of products (creams and liquids) are available nowadays that anesthetize the tissues. Drops used for the eyelids come in "single doses," i.e., in individual sterile measures. In some countries, local anesthetics are freely available, while in others a doctor's prescription is required.

Local anesthetic by injection

When it comes to carrying out permanent makeup on the lips, some clients worry that even the strongest of the mild local anesthetics will not be sufficient. If this were the case, it would be better to make an appointment with a dentist so that he can administer a local anesthetic by injection. Contrary to what is sometimes believed, this does not necessarily entail an over-saturation of the tissues with the anesthetizing liquid and a subsequent reduction in the efficiency of the pigment.

If you are not allergic to adrenaline, then lidocaine with a 1,000,000th solution of epinephrine will act as a vasoconstrictor, thus reducing the possibility of swelling and bleeding as well as prolonging the effect of the anesthetic.

Alternatively, you could ask your dentist to perform a "nerve block," thereby deadening the surrounding area. This method prevents swelling and any distortion of the tissue. The disadvantage is that the patient does not benefit from the vasoconstrictor effect.

Analgesics and sedatives

The efficacy of the products can be further reinforced with a sedative or analgesic. If this is felt necessary it can be obtained by prescription and taken just before the treatment. It might be wise to try the sedative out a few days before to check that there are no side effects.

General anesthetic

This is not necessary in permanent makeup. However, if the patient is to be given a general anesthetic, for example during an operation for breast reconstruction, it is possible to take advantage of the situation in order to pigment an areola.

I firmly believe it is the professional technician's responsibility, after discussing the subject with her client and drawing on past experience, to advise the client to visit a doctor or dentist prior to treatment so that she can be given an anesthetic. The choice of anesthetic would depend on the patient's sensitivity, how long the procedure was likely to take, etc.

Chapter XIII

Is Allergy Testing Necessary?

This is a much-debated question, not only in the field of permanent makeup but also in that of tattooing. One might think that a local skin test would soon confirm whether or not a client was allergic to the pigment and that tattooing could then proceed. Unfortunately, things are never that simple. Various aspects of the problem need to be examined.

First of all, the risks of an allergic reaction are extremely slim. Tattooing has been practiced since time immemorial and the number of scientifically recorded allergic reactions is negligible.

What factors do we need to consider in order to determine the reliability and therefore the value of such a test?

The time factor

An allergic reaction may of course manifest itself immediately. However, it can also take *months, sometimes years.* One could not expect a client to spend most of her life in the practitioner's waiting room waiting for a possible allergic reaction!

The "trigger" factor

This dreaded reaction might not take place, for some allergic reactions only manifest themselves *after prolonged exposure to the sun* (which is actually why, if a skin test is carried out, it should be done on a part of the body exposed to daylight). Moreover, an allergic reaction might not take place the first time, but rather the *second time* the skin comes into contact with the substance.

Finding the "guilty" party

Should an allergic reaction take place, it must be remembered that pigment is often made up of a mixture of several colors, and that each of these is made up of different substances. So to *which* of these is the patient reacting? However, if an allergic reaction does take place, one could begin by pointing the finger at the red pigment, before moving on to the green, blue, violet, yellow, or even black.

The personal factor

We know of several cases where a person who has never had the slightest allergic reaction to a particular substance suddenly becomes, without apparent reason, sensitive to this substance.

So, what's to be done? Personally, I believe these tests are not particularly reliable. Their great weakness is that, when there is no relatively rapid "response," they lull one into a false sense of security— and there is still no guarantee that one day the person will not have a reaction to the pigment in question.

However, if the client or technician feels that a scratch test would be beneficial, it should be carried out on an area of the body normally exposed to daylight, such as the scalp. If this is not possible, test an area that is warm and humid, such as the back of the earlobe or between the toes. It is in these highly sensitive areas of the body that a reaction is most likely to take place. And if it does, it will be in the form of pruritis (persistent itchiness) and skin eruptions (bright red rash).

In the end, having been fully informed of the facts, it is up to each individual technician to decide whether or not to perform an allergy test. After all, each of us is free to choose — when in full knowledge of the facts — our own standards of safety.

> **Warning!** Many of the photos in the following chapters were taken before and immediately after permanent makeup, which accounts for the redness and/or signs of mild swelling.
>
> The colors in these photographs can appear very distinct, dark, and intense, but after four to six days the pigmentation flakes or peels to become lighter and softer (it will lighten still further before stabilizing at the end of one month).
>
> None of these photos have been touched up.

Chapter XIV

Eyebrows

The joyful spirit always
Carries its eyebrows high…
—Pierre de Ronsard

My wife […]
with her rim of a swallow's nest eyebrows…
—André Breton, l'Union libre

The shape of the eyebrow is never straightforward. Any caricaturist will tell you this, for it is basically through the eyebrows that they vary a character's facial expressions. Raised, the eyebrows express amazement or admiration. Knit, they warn we are deep in thought or growing impatient. Thick eyebrows express strength and determination while non-existent or thin eyebrows give the impression that a person is self-effacing.

Beautiful eyebrows bring "a smile to the eye" and a particular glow to the upper part of the face. They emphasize the curvature of the brow, the depth of the pupil, and the height of the cheekbones. Permanent makeup can create a "lifting effect" by raising the drooping arch of an eyebrow, which can make a person look sad, tired, or old.

Often neglected — indeed ignored — even by well-groomed women, the eyebrows deserve as much care and attention as the eyes and mouth, because of their ability to create an atmosphere for the face.

We need to look after these mood ambassadors of ours and find out what suits them best.

Permanent makeup can embellish eyebrows by bringing out their natural line or by dressing them up, but not with a view to disguising them completely, as this might upset the face's natural harmony.

Why have your eyebrows tattooed?

✓ *Sparse or thin eyebrows.* Nature, whatever we might say about her, does not always do things well. A blunder on her part can result in imperfect, untidy eyebrows
✓ *Eyebrows too fair.* The downside for blondes is that eyebrows can become quite colorless
✓ *Eyebrows broken by a scar*
✓ *(Partial) alopecia*

- ✓ *Badly positioned or asymmetrical eyebrows*
- ✓ *Eyebrows too low or drooping*, making the person look sad, tired, or old
- ✓ *Patchy or swirling eyebrows*
- ✓ *Insufficient eyebrows* (too short)
- ✓ *Lack of eyebrow.* Fashion has at times driven many women to have their eyebrows partially or completely tweezed – a style not always easy to carry off. It is possible that the eyebrows never grow back or do not grow back properly
- ✓ *Eyebrows damaged by chemotherapy*
- ✓ *Last but not least: for pure, unadulterated pleasure.*

Symmetry and balance

Without wanting to ruffle anyone's feathers, it must be said that very few faces are symmetrical. The ears, for example, are not always level with one another; just ask your optician, who might have had to adjust your frames, ever so slightly, to compensate for the difference. You'll see that he wasn't blind to this fact!

Even if the ears are symmetrical, the face always has asymmetries that give it its individual personality. This is particularly so when it comes to the eyebrows.

Try the following experiment: place a mirror vertically to the middle of a portrait so that the face reflected in the mirror is composed of two right or two left halves…uncanny, isn't it? This is why, much of the time, it is not a case of drawing two absolutely identical eyebrows.

If you are not sure which of two diametrically opposed effects to go for, I would suggest you try out your new eyebrows beforehand. Draw them in with a cosmetic pencil and change the line every day. Instinct will eventually tell you which eyebrow shape best suits you.

Choice of line

When it comes to choosing the eyebrow line, it is important to consider the shape of the face. The actual design of the eyebrows is crucial to facial expressions. Depending on our eyebrow shape, we can look serene, sad, astonished, haughty, anxious, wise, petulant, touchy, tired, etc.

 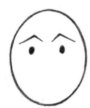 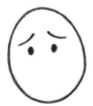 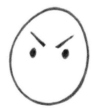 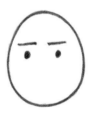

Line and physiognomy

- ✓ Curved eyebrows can soften an *angular* face (especially at the inner end, next to the top of the nose)
- ✓ On the other hand, a *softer* face can become more expressive if the eyebrows are given a more distinctive shape, e.g. like a "bird's wing"
- ✓ If the upper part of the face is *narrow*, the eyebrows can be separated and/or lengthened towards the temples in order to "widen" brow and eyes
- ✓ Conversely, a face that is too *wide* can be "slimmed down" by bringing the eyebrows closer together and/or shortening them.

The method

There are two ways of tattooing the eyebrows:

1. Hair by hair   2. Shading

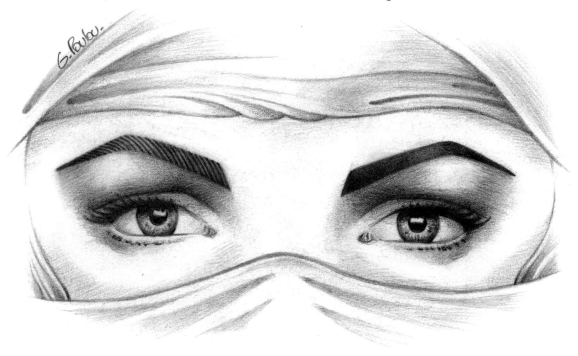

✓   Hair by hair (1)

The hair by hair method creates a more subtle effect. It makes your eyebrows look more attractive without anyone being aware of the deception. Your face will just look more harmonious.

✓   Shading (2)

Similar to a cosmetic pencil line, the resulting "powdery" effect is, without looking "conspicuous," more natural.

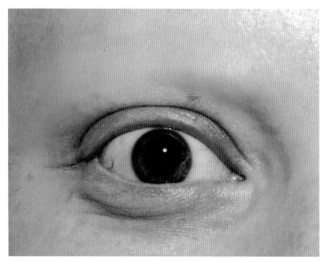
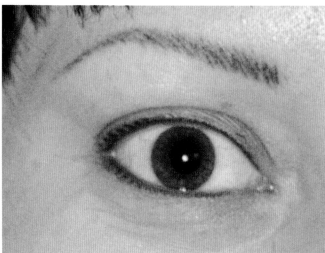

Alopecia Universalis client with hairstroke eyebrows and tattooed eyelashes. *Courtesy of Jeffery Lyle Segal (Chicago, IL and Beverly Hills, CA).*

Deciding which of the two techniques is right for each individual client must be approached with caution. Technician and client discuss the client's requirements. Using a cosmetic pencil, the technician draws the various proposals on the arches of the client's eyebrows, until both parties are satisfied with the results. There are many parameters to be taken into consideration: length, thickness, color, etc.

We frequently combine the two techniques, either to produce a soft, light background (shading), on which we draw a few darker hairs, or we draw a few hairs at the beginning of the eyebrows and work our way towards the end, drawing the hairs closer together and shading the end.

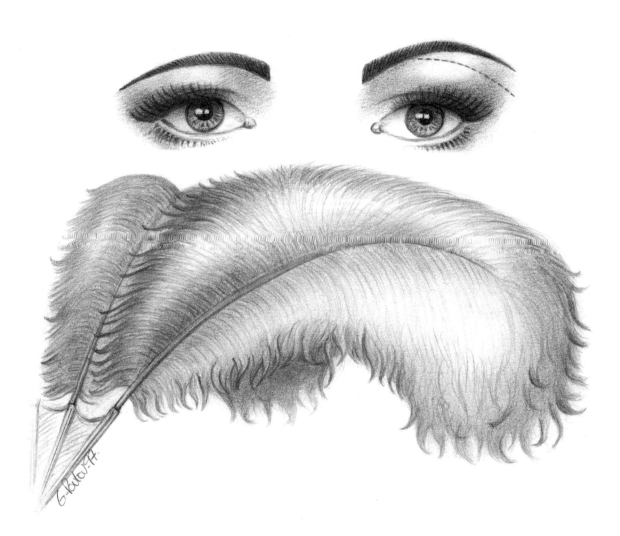

Lifting the eyebrow tail

How do we alter, as subtly and effectively as possible, the line of the eyebrow when the end (or "tail") drops slightly to create a listless, resigned expression?

All we do is pluck the eyebrow tail and then redraw it a little higher up, so as to "widen the eyes" and make them look more youthful.

Choice of color

As far as possible, go for your natural hair color, even if you dye your hair. Who can say whether you might want to change it some day — after all, isn't it a woman's prerogative to change her mind?

Eyebrow color can be lighter or darker than your hair.

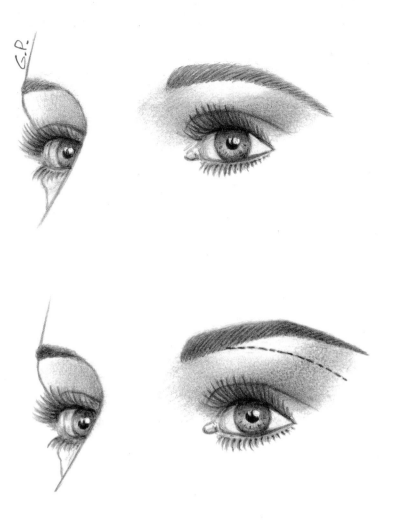

The effect of lifting eyebrow tails is quite spectacular.

We have lift-off!

Some people have just *one* eyebrow that seems to "lift off" whenever they are thinking or talking. We always point this out to a client, so that she does not come back some time later to complain that her eyebrows are not level. She will either feel that this is part of her charm and accept it, or she will ask us to "cheat" by slightly altering the position of one eyebrow.

As Inès de la Fressange so beautifully puts it: "*Beauty is often the result of a flaw. Personality is created by the breaking point.*" There have, in fact, always been two approaches to beauty. In the first a particular feature is exploited because it makes the person more attractive. And in the second a particular feature is "expunged" in an attempt to achieve a certain "purity."

Anything else?

✓ Your eyebrow must suit your face. Don't forget that not only can your physiognomy be modi-fied, but it can also be radically changed — and for a long time! Ask yourself whether your present state of mind might not have turned your head — just a little.

✓ Do you just want a change of image because you want to break with the past? Your hair-dresser will be well aware of this situation.

These observations are valid not only when it comes to permanent makeup but also with tattoos! Whatever you decide: no matter the face, no matter the beauty, well-groomed eyebrows are an asset!

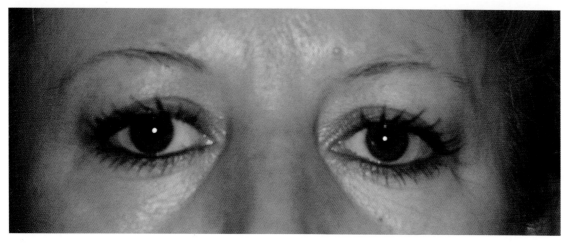

Sparse eyebrows.

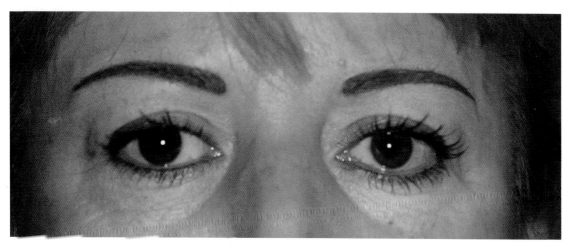

Immediately after permanent makeup. The color will become lighter and softer after a week.

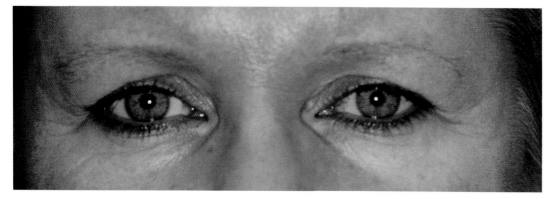

Eyebrows too fair and colorless.

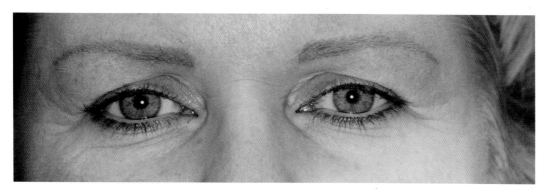

After permanent makeup.

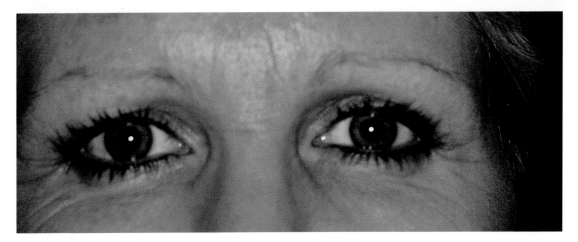

Sparse and drooping eyebrows.

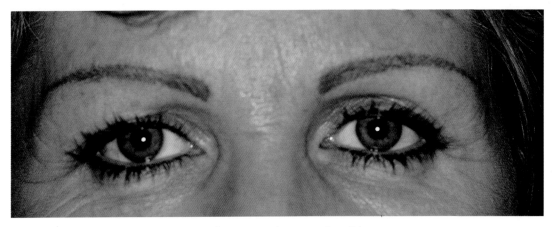

Immediately after receiving permanent makeup on eyebrows and eyelids.

Alopecia of the
eyebrows and eyelids.

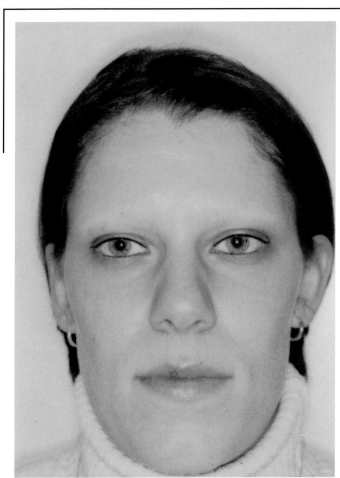

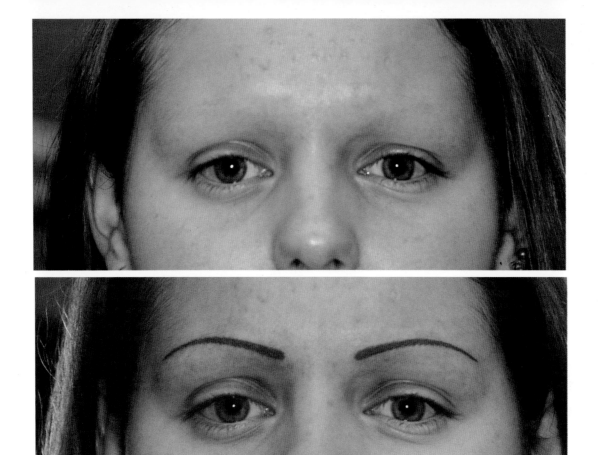

Creating permanent eyebrows on a young woman who had none.

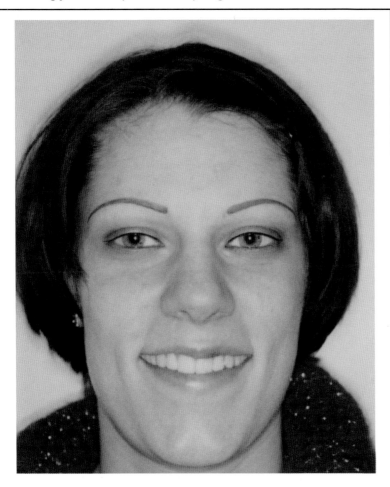

After permanent makeup.

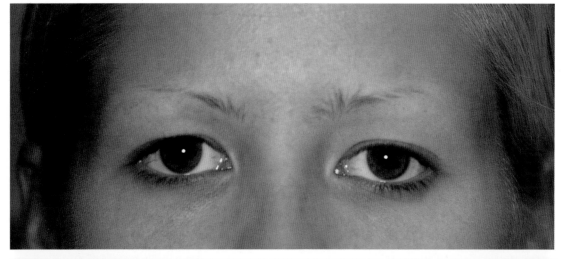

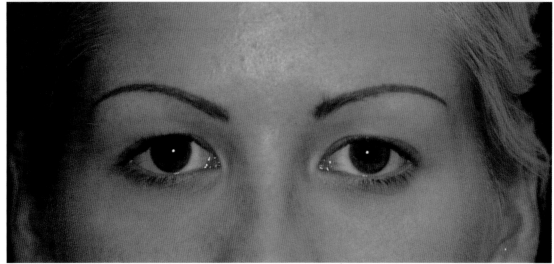

Enhancing sparse eyebrows with permanent cosmetics.

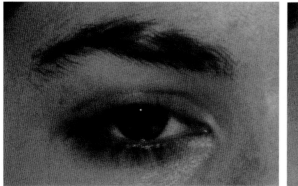 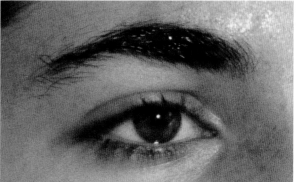

Scar camouflage in eyebrow.

68

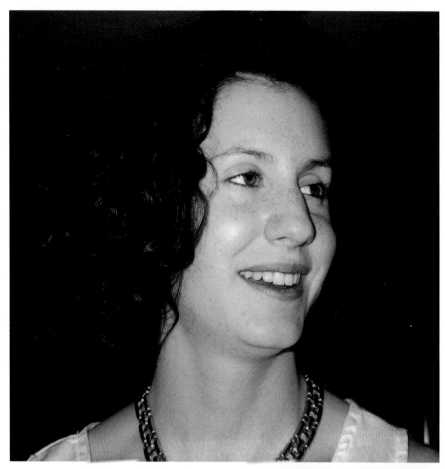

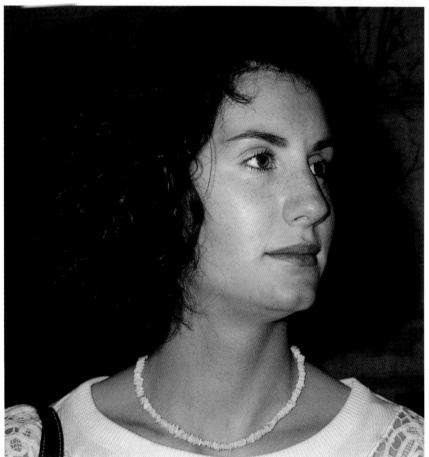

Discreet thickening of the eyebrows. *Courtesy of Institut Marion Satigny – Genève.*

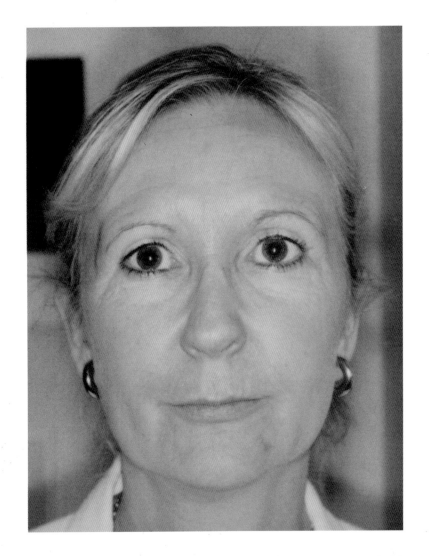

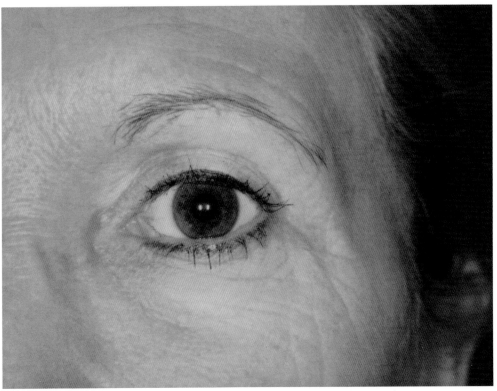

Drooping eyebrows.

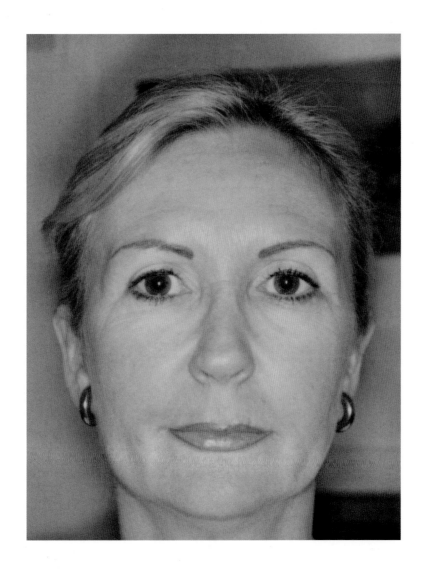

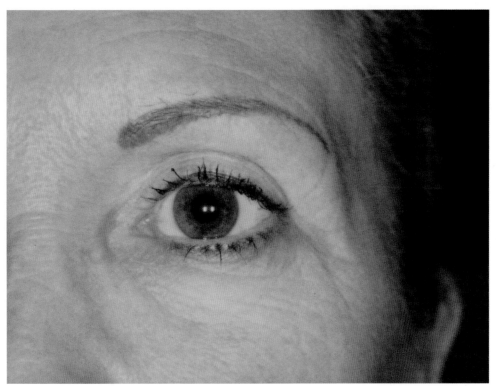

Lifting the eyebrows, along with permanent lipliner, gives this woman a more attractive and younger face.

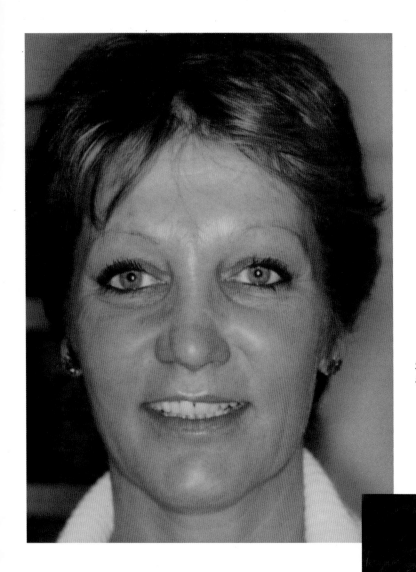

Sparse and thin eyebrows
after too much tweezing.

Immediately after receiving permanent makeup
of the eyebrows and lipliner. The color will
become lighter and softer after a week.

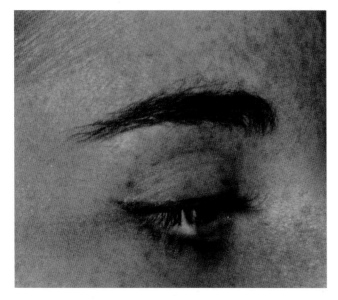

Eyebrows too short.

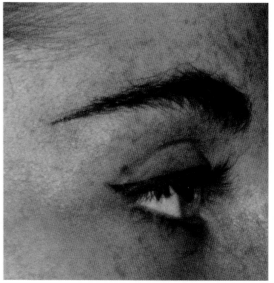

Extended eyebrow tail + permanent upper eyeliner. *Courtesy of Institut Marion, Satigny – Genève.*

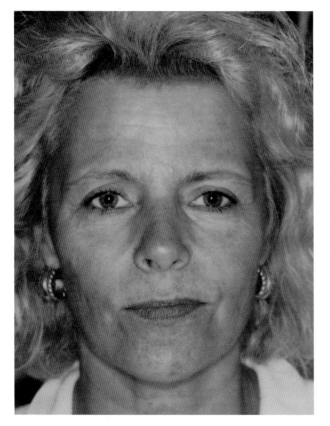

Eyebrows too low.

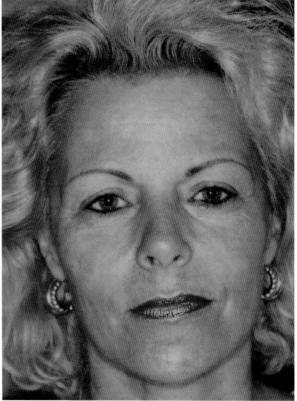

A more attractive face after raising the eyebrows and tattooing the eyeliner (just after).

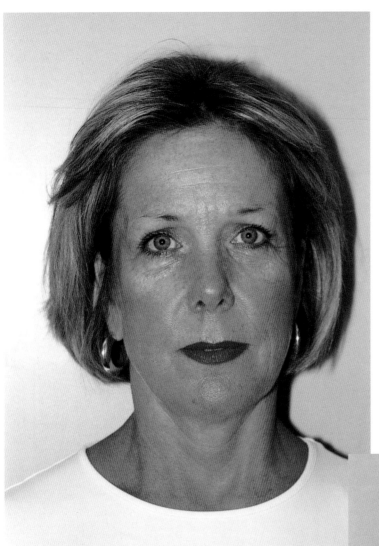

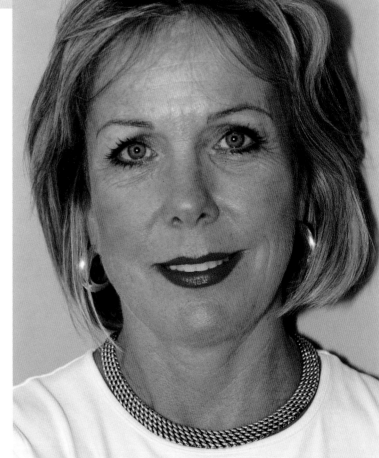

Partial brows completed with permanent makeup make this client's eyes look younger, stronger, and more beautiful. *Courtesy of Jeffery Lyle Segal (Chicago, IL and Beverly Hills, CA).*

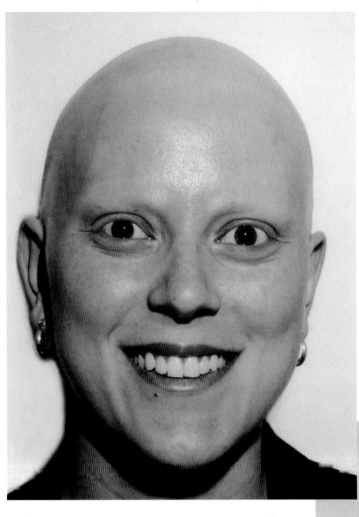

Alopecia Universalis client with hairstroke eyebrows and tattooed eyelashes. *Courtesy of Jeffery Lyle Segal (Chicago, IL and Beverly Hills, CA).*

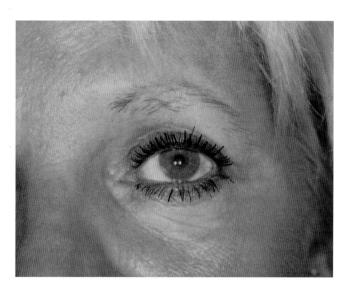

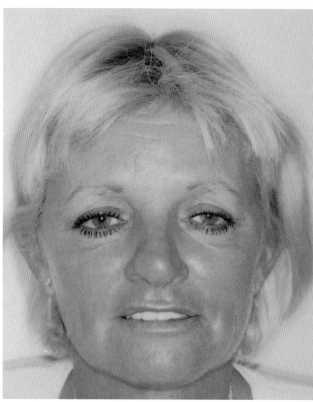

Low and drooping eyebrows.

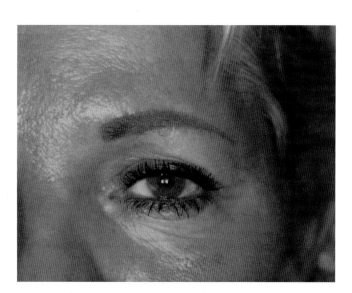

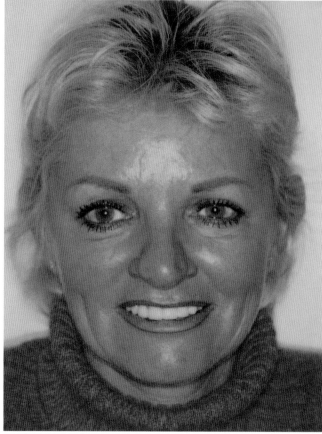

Permanent makeup gives a more radiant and younger face after lifting the eyebrows and adding permanent lipliner.

Chapter XV

Eyes

For I have to captivate these gentle lovers
Pure mirrors that make all things more beauteous
My eyes, my huge eyes with their eternal clearness
—Charles Baudelaire, *Beauty*

Your eyes are the envy of the sky after the rain…
—Louis Aragon, *Elsa's Eyes*

Since the dawn of civilization, it has been accepted that the eye is the symbol of a beginning and that it is therefore at the very heart of all things human, in other words: the soul and spirit. The first letter of both the Greek and Latin alphabets resembles an eye. It also has significance in Hebrew.

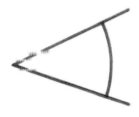

Ancient and first letter of the Greek and Latin alphabets, "A" was originally drawn on its side and resembled an eye in profile.

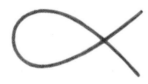

First lower case character of the Greek alphabet "alpha": the shape of the eye is unmistakable.

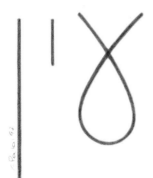

The handwritten Hebrew word for eye: "Ayin" which begins (on the right) with the letter "ayin," featuring…an eye.

The magic of the eyes — for good and bad (e.g. the "evil eye") — is quite extraordinary. "To protect themselves from the Devil, people from many different cultures were in the habit of wearing a talisman depicting an eye. A protective eye was sometimes tattooed onto a baby's back, in case the Devil sneaked up from behind…"[1]

What has not been said about the eyes! They have been likened to landscapes, stormy skies, and bottomless lakes, and referred to as the gateway to the dream world, the windows to the soul. The way they shine. The way they ensnare. They wield the same power as beauty and seduction. One of the most famous lines in French cinema is when Jean Gabin says to Michèle Morgan: "You got beautiful eyes, you know…"[2]

Eyes also betray our emotions. We might not always realize it, but their power to persuade depends on how expressive they are. To prevent them from giving too much away, we sometimes avert our gaze or lower our eyes. And, since time immemorial, we have used makeup to set off our eyes by applying eyeliner or a kohl-line. To show a painting to its best advantage, we frame it. In much the same way we "dress" our eyes with *eyeliner* and *a kohl-line*. Our eyes become more expressive, deeper.

Nowadays, this type of makeup is usually used only by women. This has not always been the case, however. In the seventeenth century, John Bulwer wrote: "The Turks have a black powder made of a mineral called alchole[3] which they apply below the eyelids with a fine brush, thus darkening them and thereby emphasizing the whites of their eyes. They also use this powder to dye their lashes. It is the women in particular who do this." He goes on to say that "Xenephon described how the Mèdes were in the habit of applying makeup to their eyes."

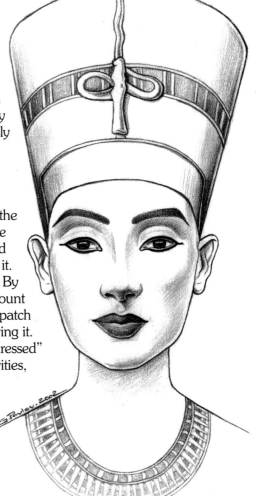

We have discovered, from paintings and sculptures that date back to ancient Egypt, that men as well as women were in the habit of applying makeup to their eyes and eyebrows. The whole of the eye was outlined. This line and the eyebrow line were extended over onto the temple. Queen Nefertiti reigned some thirty-five centuries ago, but who can see pictures of her face and not find her striking beauty and truly contemporary look fascinating? She obviously had already perfected of the art of applying makeup.

Why go in for permanently made-up eyes?

However perfect the lines you draw at seven in the morning, your work of art will rapidly become "smudged" due to the combined action of blinking and the moistness of the eyeball. It smears. It runs. You fix it. It smears again. The cycle repeats several times a day. By eleven o'clock at night, your heart sinks: despite the amount that has already come off, and despite your attempts to patch it up, you are still confronted with the chore of removing it.

Apart from the wish to have permanently "well-dressed" eyes and the wish to avoid similar time-wasting activities, what are the reasons for having your eyelids tattooed?

✓ Your lashes are too fair
✓ You have sparse or missing lashes
✓ Your eyes frequently water in the wind, cold, light, and when you are ill
✓ You suffer from dry eyes
✓ You cannot see what you are doing without glasses

Queen Nefertiti

✓ Your hand is not always steady
✓ You wear contact lenses and your optician has quite rightly advised you not to put them in until you have finished applying your makeup
✓ In any case, the less you torture your eyes with a pencil, the better it is for them...

Here are the various options:

✓ **Lash-Liner**

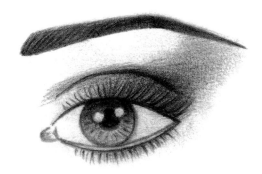

This entails the tattooing of tiny dots between the lashes. Each dot imitates a growing eyelash. The intention — to give the impression that the person has more eyelashes — has the advantage of following a line that is never affected by the vagaries of fashion: the lash-bearing rim of the eyelid.

The upper lid has between 70 and 160 lashes and the under lid between 70 and 80. They do not turn white with age and have a life span of three to five months before falling out and being replaced. What more attractive accent than beautiful lashes could you have for your eyes?

The lash-liner is the ideal solution for those who wish to look as natural as possible.

✓ **Eyeliner**

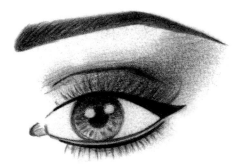

Whether it is applied above or below your eyes, this line is destined to make them look larger.

There are countless women who want to have "almond-shaped" eyes by having the tattooed eyeliner extended outwards. Asian women, on the other hand, want their eyes to look more "rounded" and have the line thicker at the center.

Upper eyeliner

A *discreet*, silky effect can be achieved by partially or completely "thickening" the natural fringe, without going beyond either the first or the last lash.

To create an *almond-shaped eye*, the beginning of the line is thin and is gradually thickened towards the temple, where it can be extended with a small "wing" or "tail." The length and thickness of the line can be varied depending on the size and shape of the eye.

Lower eyeliner

For a *discreet* effect, the same method as used for the upper lid can be applied to the under lid.

For *almond-shaped eyes*, we avoid accentuating the "U"-shape of the under lid on people with very "rounded" eyes. To achieve a straighter line, at each end of the eye, we move slightly away from the line formed by the eyelash fringe. Here too the line is thin at the beginning and can, if desired, be gradually thickened towards the end.

It should be pointed out that to join upper and lower eyeliner at the outside corner of the eye would create the illusion that the eye was "closing." Moreover, as the skin is this area is very delicate, there is also the risk that the pigment might spread during pigmentation into a particularly unattractive "flame of color."

✓ The kohl-line

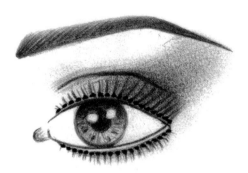

"Kohl me": here is a cry that cannot be ignored…conjuring images of the Orient and the *eyes of the beautiful Scheherazade*, storyteller of genius (and of genies), who held the King of Persia spellbound for One Thousand and One Nights.

The origin of kohl has been lost in the mists of time. It would appear that as well as sublimating the eyes it was originally used as an eye treatment. The preparation was made from antimony, an extremely hard mineral that was crushed and pounded by hand before being mixed with a vegetable cocktail, such as musk, cloves, and date stones. The kohl-line was applied to the flat edge of the eyelid, to the area situated between the eyeball and the lashes. It emphasized the white of the eye, giving depth to the gaze. It is not recommended for people keen to enlarge their eyes since it has quite the opposite effect.

Unlike eyeliner, the kohl-line is in constant contact with the saline solution we call tears; this has a "blanching" effect. The speed with which it "fades" depends very much on the eye's level of salinity[4].

✓ A combination of styles

It is of course possible to combine all three styles. For example, the eyeliner dots can gradually be brought closer together so that the line becomes stronger the closer it gets to the temple. Similarly, it is not unusual to add a kohl-line to eyeliner or vice versa.

As a result of the lachrymal glands being stimulated by the procedure, the eyelids can become slightly swollen (as happens when we cry) due to water retention. The effect can last for between twenty-four and forty-eight hours. A homeopathic remedy can relieve the symptoms. It is recommended that a mixture of *Arnica* and *Ledum 20c* be taken eight to twelve hours prior to and following the procedure. Cold compresses are also helpful, the most effective being the small sachets (previously placed in the freezer) that contain a cold-retaining blue fluid.

If you wear contact lenses, you should bring a pair of prescription glasses with you; it is advisable not to wear contact lenses immediately after permanent makeup, for the simple reason that:

✓ the eye is still numb from the anesthetic and you risk damaging the cornea, as you cannot feel what you are doing

✓ there might still be particles of pigment on the surface of the eye which, although invisible, might become trapped under the lens, as the eye would be unable to clean itself naturally.

Admittedly we are reluctant to touch the area of the eyelids, but experience has shown that they are less sensitive than is generally thought. Don't worry, your eyeliner won't become "ow-liner"! We are careful to numb your lids. You won't feel a thing.

What wouldn't I do for your beautiful eyes?

[1]Desmond Morris, *Body Watching/Talk*.
[2]Marcel Carné: *Port of Shadows*.
[3]Hence the modern term "kohl." This text comes from the facsimile of Bulwer's work in Desmond Morris, *ibid*.
[4]It is said that sailors used to "blanch" tattoos they no longer cared for by soaking their forearms in seawater for as long and as often as possible.

Questions for the expert

An Interview with *Dr. Bernard Hayot, Paris, France*
Cosmetic Laser Surgery

If I have my eyelids tattooed, do I run the risk of permanently losing my eyelashes?

You can only lose your eyelashes permanently when the follicle of the eyelash is destroyed. The process is known as ciliary electrolysis (a fine needle is inserted into the follicle and an electric current is passed through into the follicle thereby destroying it). Permanent removal of unwanted hair developed from this technique, discovered in 1880, by an American ophthalmologist. You cannot therefore permanently lose your lashes following dermapigmentation.

Can cosmetic surgery to the upper or under eyelids in any way degrade tattooed eyeliner?

*In the case of **lower blepharoplasty**, if the eyeliner is just below the eyelashes it might be removed because we cut away a few millimeters of surplus (and therefore tattooed) skin. There are two possible solutions to this:*

1. *To make the incision just below the eyeliner, leaving it untouched. However, the scar, 1 or 2 mm below the ciliary rim, might form a "ridge" as a result of skin adhesions.*

2. ***The best solution** would be to go for transconjunctival blepharoplasty by CO_2 laser (this cuts into the conjunctiva inside the lid and leaves no visible scarring) in conjunction with laser treatment to re-tighten the skin of the eyelid, thereby leaving the eyeliner untouched.*

*In the case of **upper blepharoplasty**, the eyeliner is in no danger, for the incision is made in the palpebral fold. We should simply point out that if the eyeliner tail is long it could end up slightly raised.*

Are there any clients who should not have an eyeliner tattooed on the eye-lid rim or a kohl-line tattooed to the flat edge of the eyelid?

Only people who suffer from acute or chronic inflammation of the ciliary rim (blepheritis).

What is your opinion of permanently made-up eyelids?

We frequently recommend eyeliner. The request usually comes from the patient herself, especially if she is a busy career woman who does not want to waste time putting on makeup every day.

We often recommend it following corrective surgery, when a scar needs to be camouflaged because it is either too far from the under lid or, being white, too obvious.

We also recommend it to patients who have had their eyebrows lifted. The technique, often used to lift the eyebrow tail (and at the same time the upper lid), leaves a scar above the eyebrow. Permanent makeup can camouflage it. Used in conjunction with one another, the two techniques produce some very satisfying results.

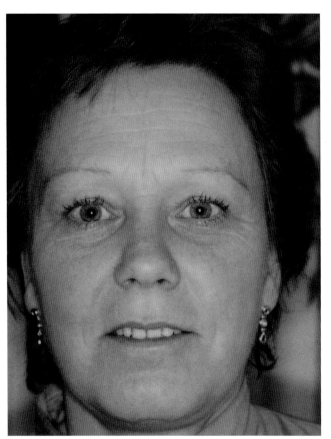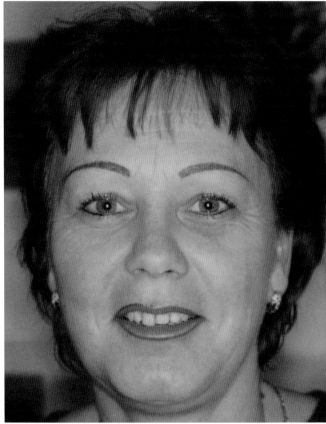

Permanent lower eyeliner adds to the sparkle already in this woman's eyes (+ permanent eyebrows and lipliner).

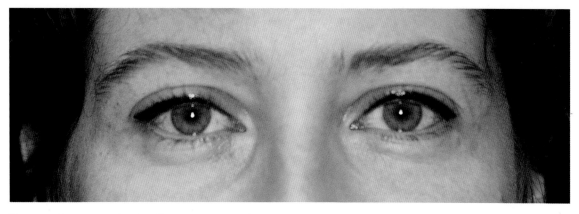

Upper eyeliner immediately after permanent makeup procedure.

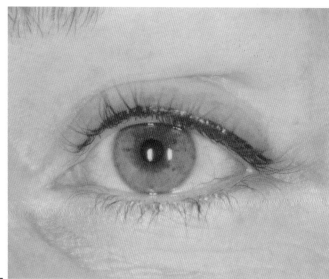

Healed upper eyeliner one week later.

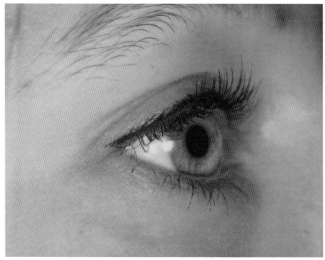

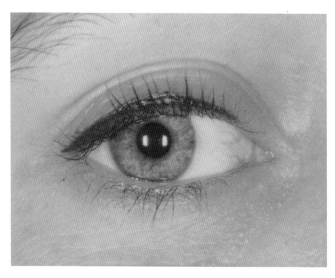

Medium thick upper eyeliner one week
after permanent makeup procedure.

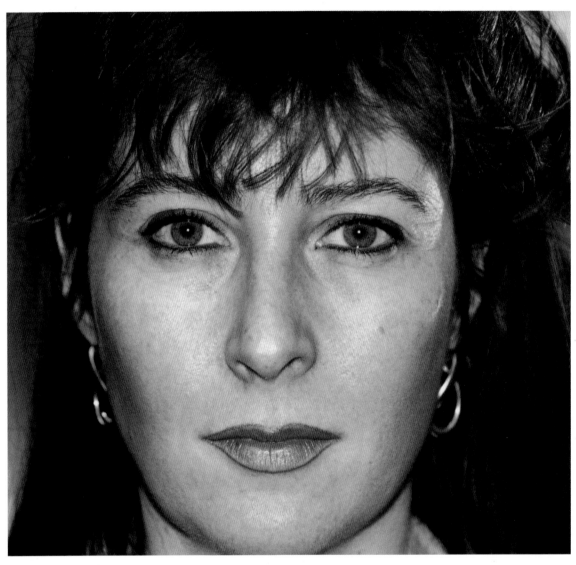

Notice how the purple upper and lower permanent eyeliner brings out the contrast of her green eyes (+ heart-shaped permanent lipliner)

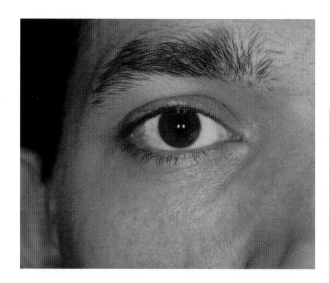

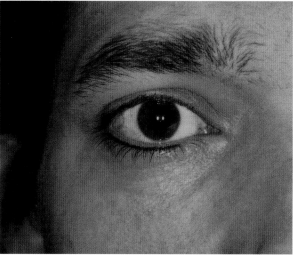

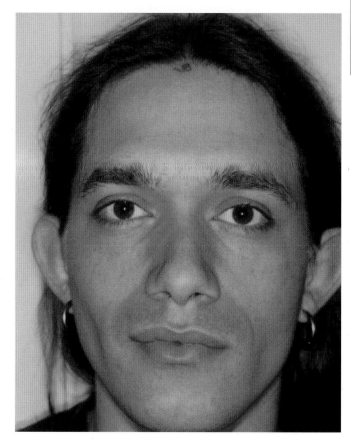

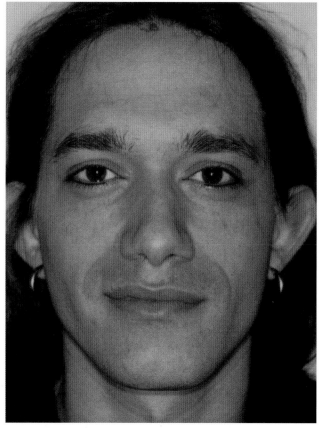

Some men also enjoy the effects of permanent
eyeliner. Immediately after procedure.

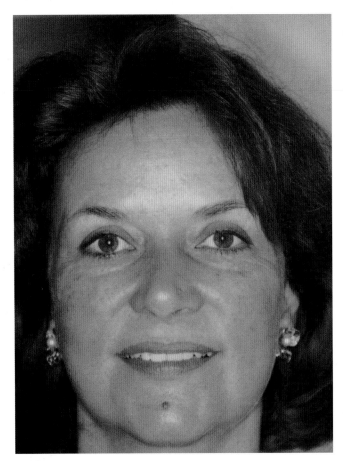
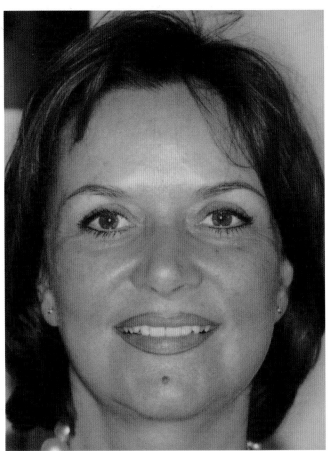

Permanent upper and lower eyeliner, eyebrows, and lipliner bring out the natural beauty of this woman's face.

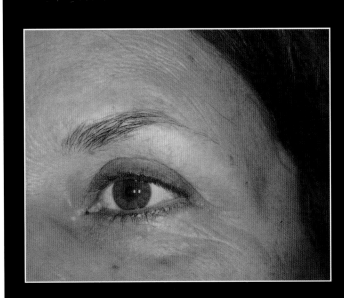
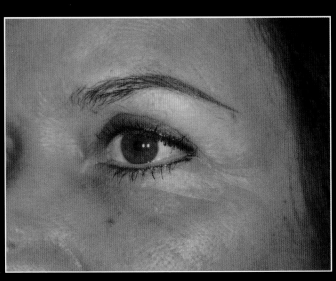

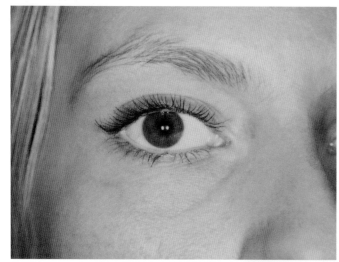

Before.

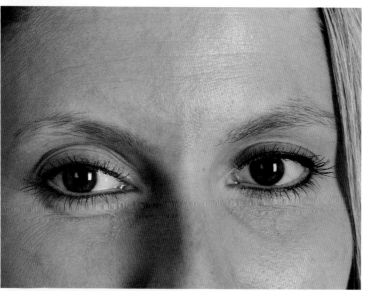

After permanent makeup.

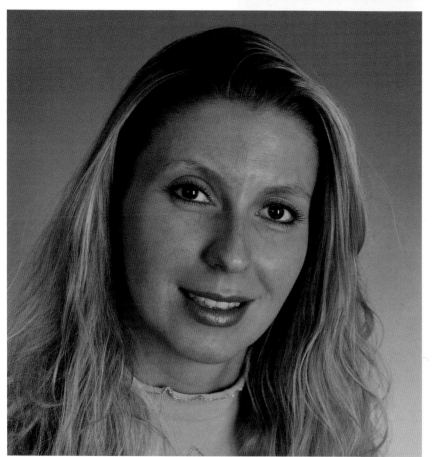

Almond shaped upper
and lower eyeliner.

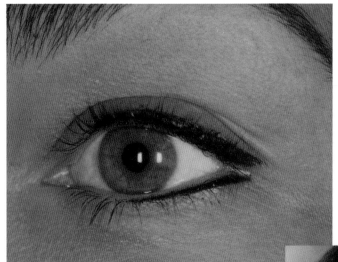

Upper and lower eyeliner immediately after tattooing give this woman…

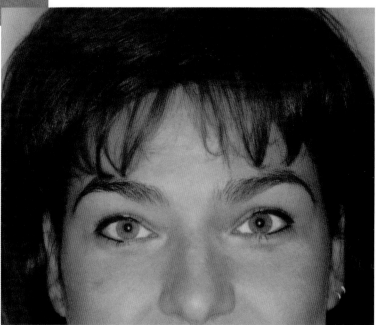

…wider and more expressive eyes.

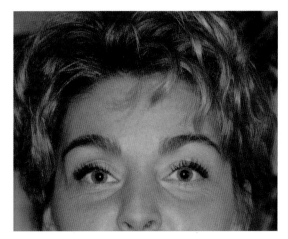

Upper eyeliner one week after tattooing…

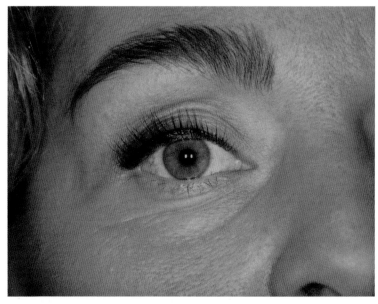

…gives more character to the eyes.

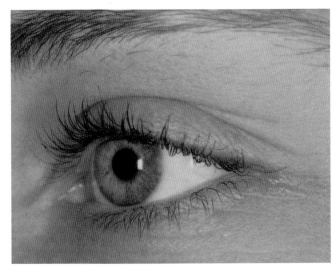

Before…

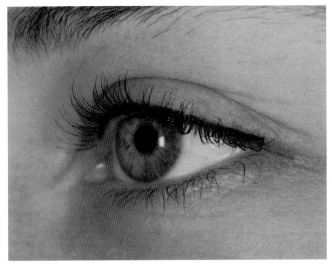

One month later.

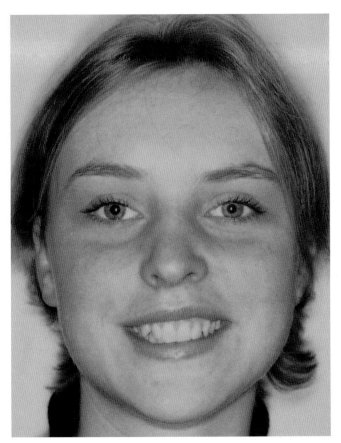

Before…

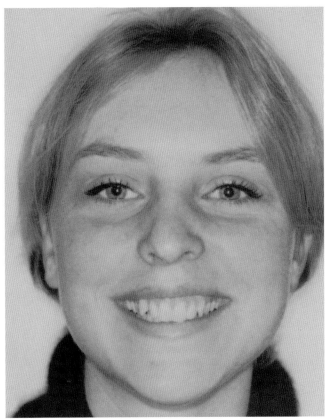

The next day.

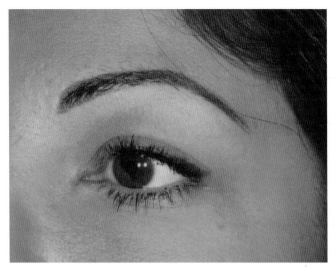

Permanently tattooed eyebrows, …

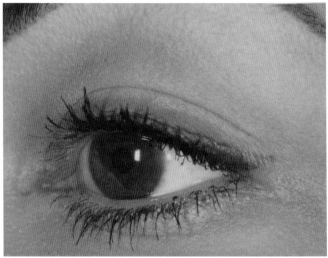

eyeliner, …

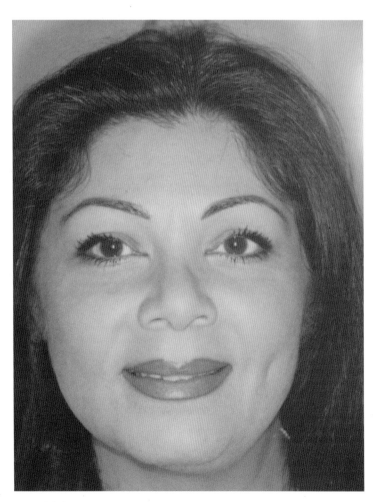

… and full lips give more character to this woman's face.

Chapter XVI

Lips

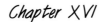

When you laugh Ninon, you know a bee
Could mistake your ruby lips for a flower
—Alfred de Musset

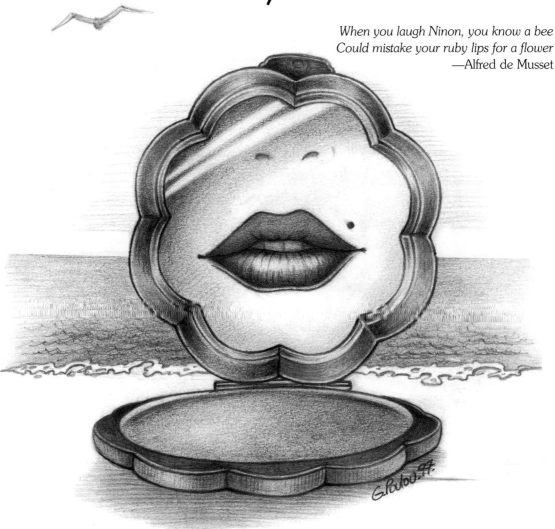

With a smile, a word, a kiss, our natural ambassadors — the lips — express our innermost state of mind and the quality of our relationships. Full, well-colored lips are the supreme symbol of femininity and the power to seduce. Women are only too well aware of this (and so are men)! It is true that puritans everywhere banned and still ban the wearing of lipstick. Is it because it is a reminder of the "forbidden fruit"?

To show their lips at their best, women have always practiced the art of makeup. It is effective, but unfortunately you have to keep reapplying it.

And, while nature has endowed some of us with a perfectly well defined mouth, others are bothered that their lips are too thin, too flat, and lacking in symmetry.

In a world that puts so much emphasis on appearance, the mouth, whether we like it or not, is seen as the face's signature. When we enhance a woman's lips with permanent makeup, we know that to her it is more than a mere detail. Her self-image is improved and this is then projected to the world at large.

Full lips are evocative of youth and a body full of vitality that yearns for the sun, fruit, and love.

Beautiful lips are an invitation. An invitation to life.

Physiology of the lips

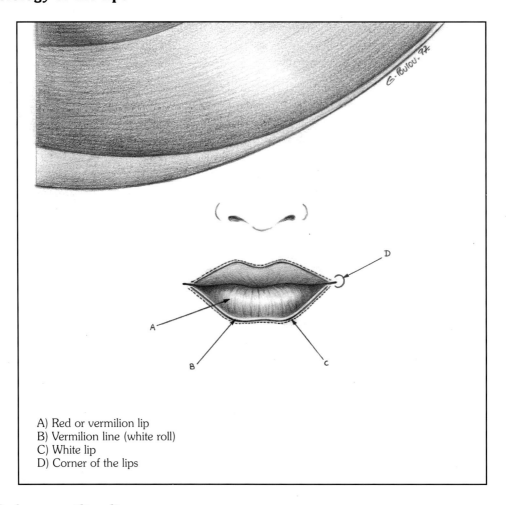

A) Red or vermilion lip
B) Vermilion line (white roll)
C) White lip
D) Corner of the lips

A) *Red or vermilion lip*

It is semi-mucous, in as much as it is an intermediary structure between skin and mucous. Retention of pigment color: around 20-50%.

B) *Vermilion line(white roll)*

It delineates the contour of the red lip, and has, in the middle of the upper lip, the very aptly named "Cupid's bow." Color retention is around 60-80%.

C) *White lip*

This area surrounds the red lips; it is a delicately structured skin that retains color to around 80-100%.

D) *Corner of lip*

These are the extremities of the mouth. Permanent makeup is not recommended, because, given the "spongy structure" of the skin, there is a risk the pigment will spread.

The lipliner

To make them look less "flat" it is often enough just to trace a line around the contour of the lips, just as we would underline a word to make it stand out. This is a relatively recent practice, at least in the West, since it would appear to have only been adopted some thirty years ago.

This is a very important line since it distinguishes the mouth from the face, making the former stand out. It can be used to correct asymmetries. It often adds a fitting touch of a color, chosen for being different from that of the red lips.

We aim above all for *balance*. The lips must always look natural (when speaking, smiling, laughing, etc.) through the interaction of light and shade. For a more "rounded" effect, we create an essentially nuanced contrast between the color of the lip contour (darker) and that of the lips themselves (lighter).

Using the interaction of light and shade to create a three-dimensional look

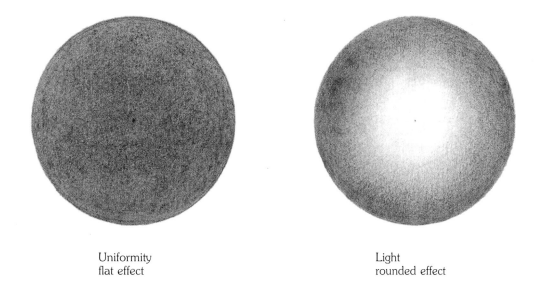

Uniformity
flat effect

Light
rounded effect

We can make the upper lip look more shapely, more rounded, by "*highlighting*" it. We "draw" a flesh-colored line (lighter than the skin tone but not white) around and just above the edge of the lip contour.

Lips come in all shapes and sizes, and there are many ways to "cheat"!

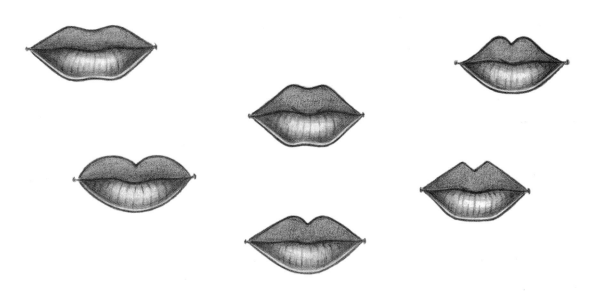

Some of the ways we can "cheat" with the lips

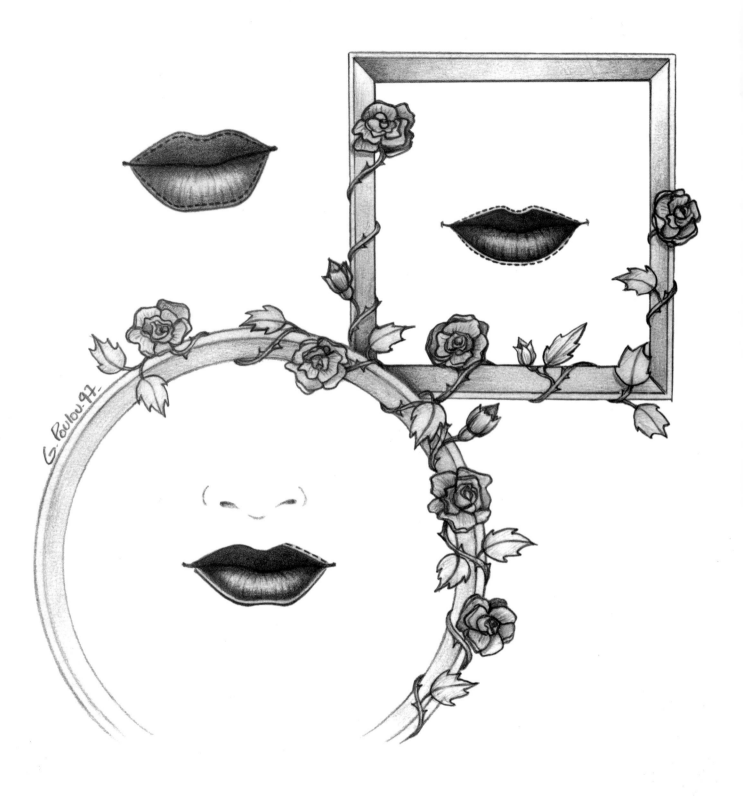

G. Poulou. 97.

A few examples

✓ A more "greedy" mouth

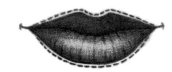

The majority of clients want their mouths to look more full. In order to achieve this, we trace a line that faithfully follows the perimeter, at a very slight but regular distance from the lips. If the distance is too great, the end result will look artificial and the opposite effect will be achieved. The mouth will look smaller but as though it is in too big a "frame." The space between contour and line can then be filled in with natural red lip color.

And what color should the line be? It must of course harmonize with skin, eyes, and hair. A stronger color will give a well-groomed, indeed sophisticated look. However, the closer it is to the lip color, the more natural it will look. There are various options and — bearing in mind the above guidelines — you can be as extravagant as you like.

✓ A more discreet mouth

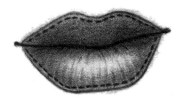

Requests for a more discreet mouth are quite rare but they can happen. We trace a line, following the perimeter of the red lip as for a "greedy mouth," but inside it. The line is thicker and the color stronger than the natural color, because the red lip only retains 20-25% of the pigment.

✓ Correction of asymmetries

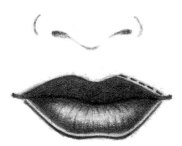

Virtually all of us have an asymmetrical mouth, which is not necessarily devoid of charm. More often than not, clients want their lips rebalanced, with a lip perimeter that "enlarges" and "corrects."

The main difficulty with this type of procedure is that the line cuts across red lip, vermilion line, and white lip. But, as the capacity to retain color by each of these skin tissues is different, it is necessary to vary the color *density* according to the tissue, so that the final line looks and remains homogenous. Furthermore, because the color of the "canvas" (red or white lip) can also change, the density as well as the *color* must vary to give a truly monochrome final line. A harmonious result will only be achieved if color is painstakingly researched.

Full lips

"Permanent lipstick" is the expression currently used to refer to this effect. Given the low color retention capacity of the texture of the red lip (20-50%), we prefer the term "veil of color." No one should be deceived into thinking the final result will look like lipstick.

However, the technique does make pale lips look more prominent in a most pleasing way. Combined with the pigmentation of the lip perimeter, it creates a more sensuous, more generous mouth.

To create this permanent "lip veil," it is absolutely essential to take into account the underlying cold color (blue-violet) of the lips, which can radically, disagreeably, and permanently change the tone selected. We abandon brown tones that have a tendency to take on a "muddy" appearance, in favor of warm, red and orange tones.

Moreover, colored lips show up the whiteness of the teeth (and smile). This is probably why men and women in Africa (and maybe elsewhere) tattoo their gums — blue/black — with soot.

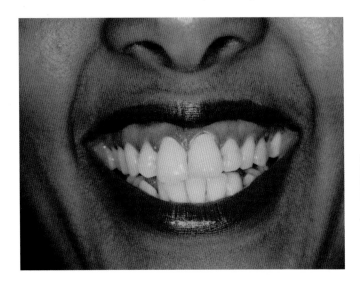

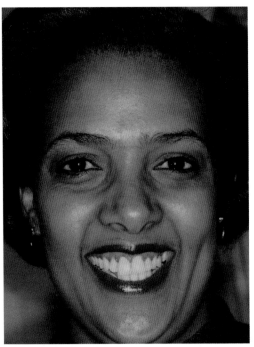

Woman with tattooed gums, a native of Oromo (Ethiopia).

The lips of Maori women

The leading exponents of the ancient art of enhancing the lips to make them more seductive are the Maori people.

These natives of New Zealand (discovered by Captain Cook in 1769) had perfected their thousand-year-old art of tattooing the faces and bodies of both men and women. Their rich and elegant tattoos were mostly colored black. The men's faces bore motifs that were usually symmetrical with their vertical axes (the nose). These motifs were very often extremely delicate spirals. At first glance it looked as though more than one person bore the same drawings. However, upon closer examination, subtle variations could be detected, which made each human being a unique work of art. And in much the same way that we protect out priceless works of art, so the Maoris preserved the most beautiful heads of their dead.

The women, on the other hand, had their lips and chins tattooed. The whole of the lips was usually tattooed black, while the chin was covered in superb geometric patterns. The upper lip was sometimes decorated with a black contour, some two to three millimeters above the vermilion.

The lip's natural red color did not seem to correspond to the Maori ideal of beauty. This is revealed in a song that used to be chanted while the young women were being tattooed. It was to calm and encourage them:

96

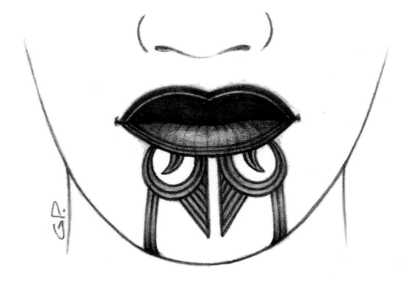

Lay thyself quietly down, oh daughter,
(soon it will be done).
That thy lips may be well tattooed;
('Tis quickly performed).
For thy going to visit the young men's houses;
Lest it be said
Whither indeed is this ugly woman going?
Now coming hitherward.
Keep thyself still, lying down, oh young lady,
(Round the tap goes).
That thy lips may be well tattooed,
Also thy chin;
That thou mayest be beautiful.
Thus it goes fast.
For thy going to visit the houses of courtship,
Lest it should be said of thee,
Whither does this woman think of going with her red lips!
"Who is walking this way?
 (Still it is revolving).
Give thyself willingly to be tattooed;
Briefly it is over.
For thy going to the house of amusement;
Also thou wilt be spoken of:
"Wither goes this woman with her bare lips,
Hastening hither, indeed, in that state?"
(Round it revolves).
It is done. It is tattooed.
(soon it is indeed).
Give hither quietly thy chin to be imprinted;
(Nimbly the hand moves).
For thy going to the houses of the single men,
Lest these words be said –
"Whither goes the woman with her red chin,
Who is coming this way"

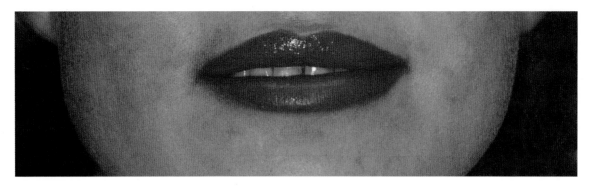

Full lips — immediately after procedure.

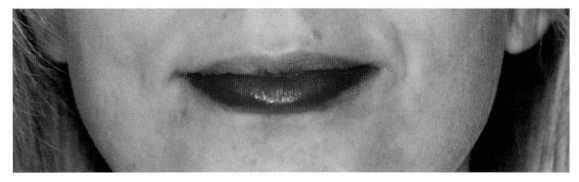

Full lower lip — immediately after procedure. Upper lip not yet begun.

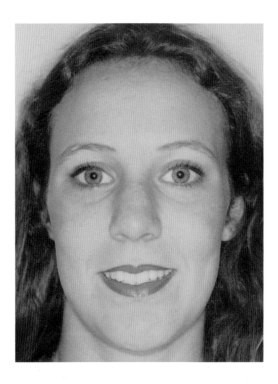

This woman received thicker lip contour and tattooed upper eyeliner.

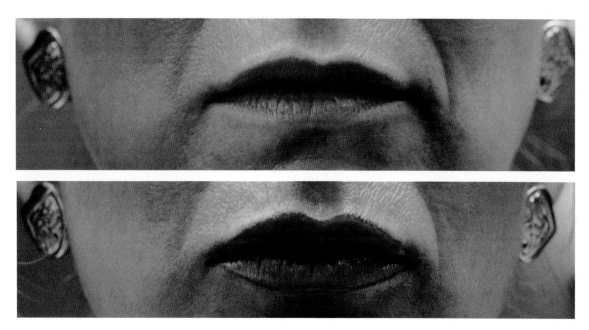

Light permanent lipliner to correct upper and lower asymmetry.

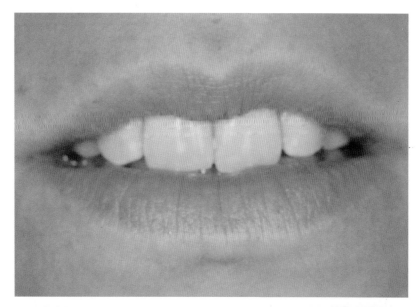

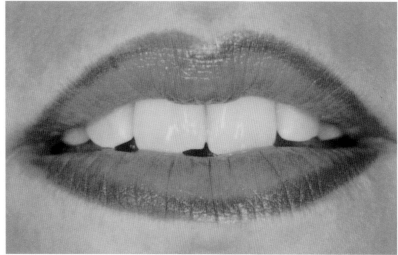

Thicker lip contour, creating a more
distinct and greater lip volume.

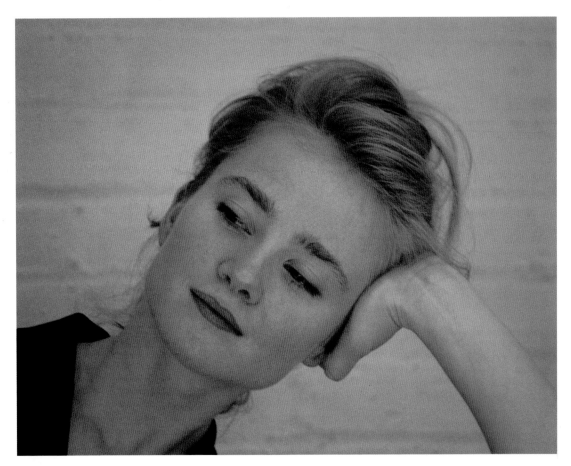

Discreet lipliner.

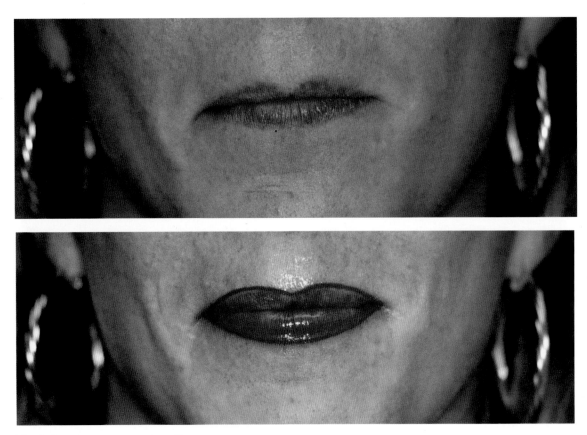

This lipliner has a rejuvenation effect.

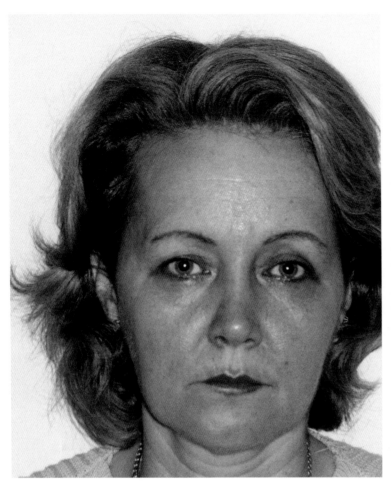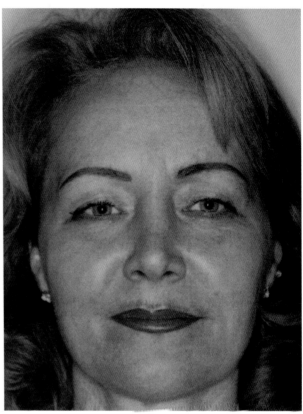

A younger looking, fuller mouth and enhanced eyebrows after receiving permanent makeup.

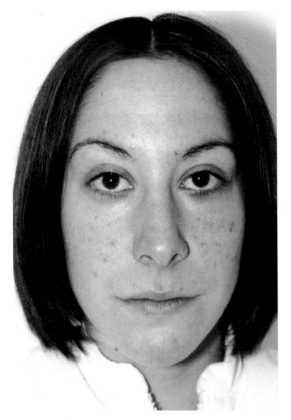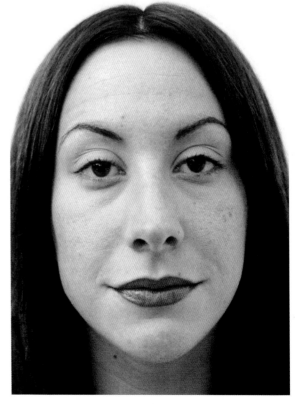

Full lip color adds definition and fullness to this client's mouth. *Courtesy of Jeffery Lyle Segal (Chicago, IL and Beverly Hills, CA).*

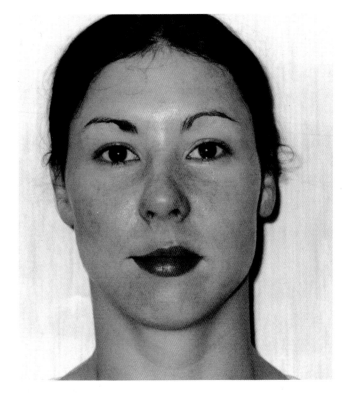

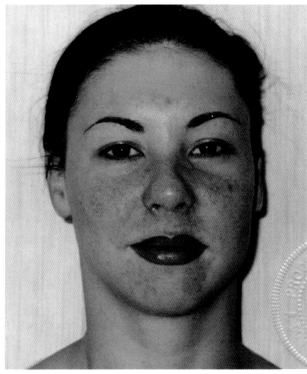

Permanent cosmetic correction of asymmetry of the upper lip. Enhancement of eyebrows and eyeliner. *Courtesy of Dominique Bossavy.*

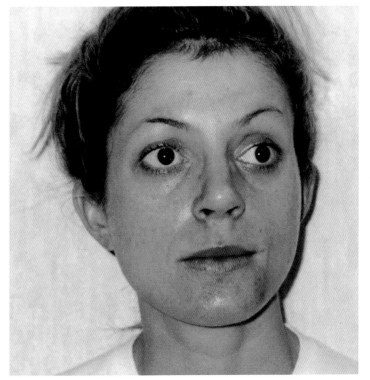

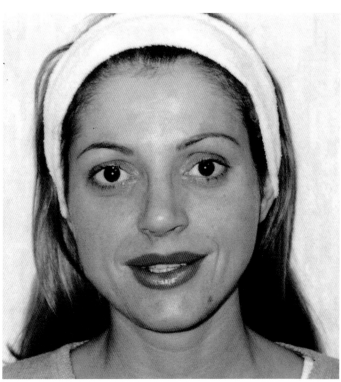

Full lips and eyebrows after permanent makeup give this woman a softer face. *Courtesy of Dominique Bossavy.*

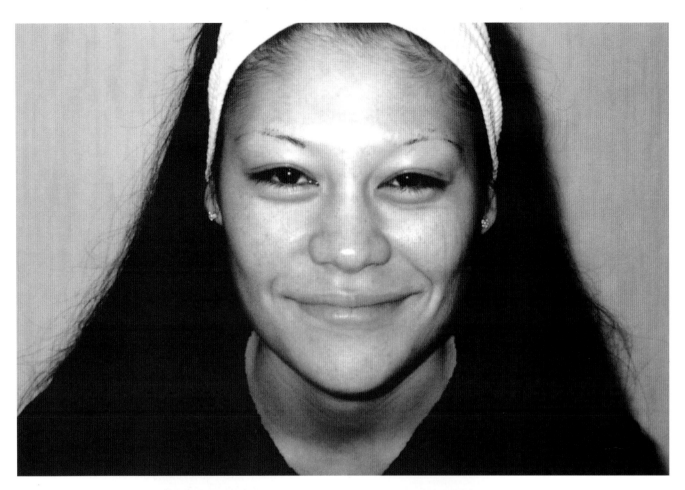

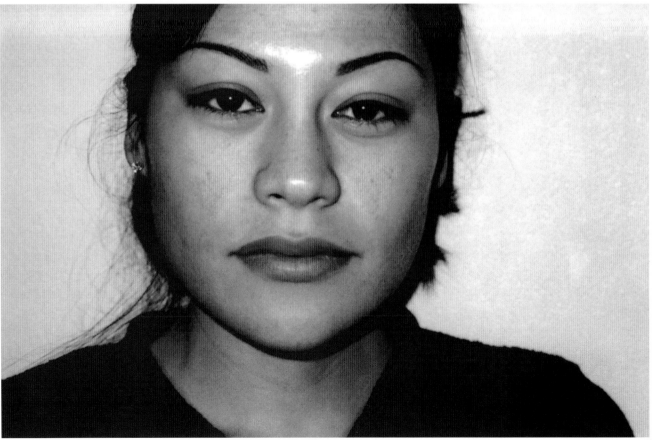

Permanent cosmetic enhancement for the lips, eyeliner, and eyebrows gives more character to this young woman's face. *Courtesy of Dominique Bossavy.*

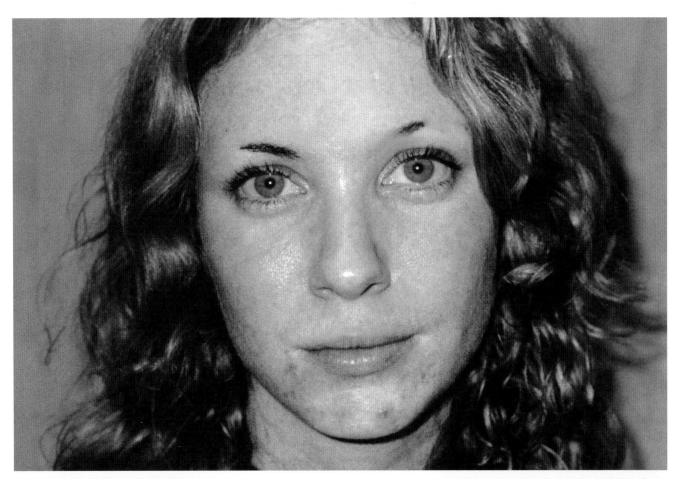

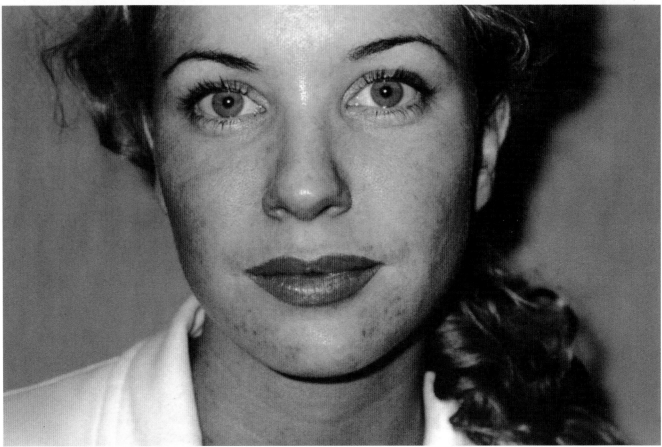

Micropigmentation of the lips and the eyebrows brings out the natural beauty of her face.
Courtesy of Dominique Bossavy.

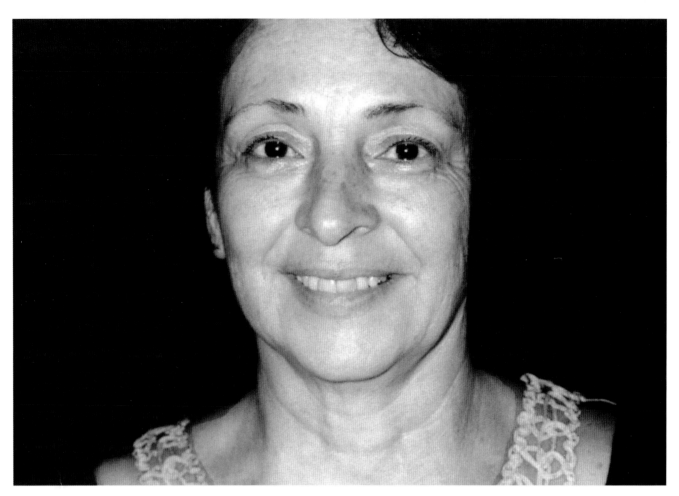

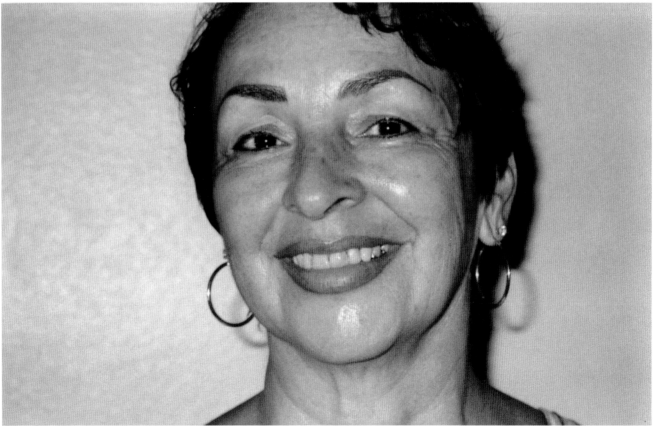

Permanent makeup brings fullness to her lips and more expression to the eyes and eyebrows.
Courtesy of Dominique Bossavy.

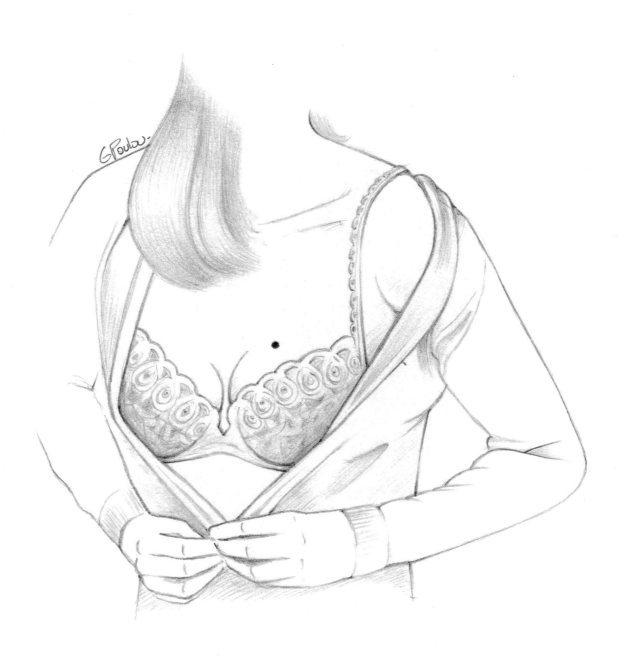

106

Chapter XVII

Beauty spot

The superfluous, a thing so necessary
—Voltaire, *Satires, Le Mondain*

The conquest of the superfluous is spiritually
more exciting than the conquest of the necessary.
—Gaston Bachelard, *La Psychanalyse du feu*

Beauty spot: so richly deserving of its name. Nature did well to create such a personal touch. But capricious as nature is, the beauty spot is not always put in the right place.

At the time of the Sun King (Louis XIV), women — particularly those at court — sought to draw attention to themselves with beauty spots (or "flies" as they were called in France at that time) placed on the face or breast. Made of a tiny velvet or taffeta disc, they accentuated the much-coveted whiteness of their skins. These "moles" (as they are also known in English) in fact go back to the time of Louis XIII and dental problems, when a patch, covered in black velvet, was applied to the cheek.

Because women were not supposed to speak of things pertaining to love, cunning little minxes that they were, they invented a whole coded language around the "mole." Where they chose to place it, had a very precise significance. The men to whom the message was destined were willing accomplices to this game.

One might at first think that permanent makeup has no role to play when it comes to beauty spots. After all, they are quick and easy enough to draw with a pencil. But are they really "natural"? It might look a little suspicious if one day a woman has an enchanting beauty spot, while the next day, it is no longer there. What a disappointment, especially to the man who adored it!

The beauty spot is ideally suited to permanent makeup, especially these days. As we no longer need to send coded messages it does not matter that it cannot be moved around.

A tattooed beauty spot actually looks more natural than one that is penciled in. On the breast, buttock, close to the navel, or wherever you fancy, it will attract attention and subtly enhance the area. It can also cleverly disguise tiny scars (from acne to chickenpox, etc.).

There are two conditions that must be respected when it comes to tattooing a beauty spot:

✓ Avoid pure black, which can produce a bluish tinge

✓ Never have an existing beauty spot tattooed. It is a known fact that in certain situations beauty spots can have adverse reactions, e.g. overexposure to the sun or, more importantly, to certain microtraumas such as tattooing.

It is often said that the beauty spot is a "trademark" (though far more charming and discernible than fingerprints), since it is never found in the same spot nor with the same characteristics as on another person. It is great fun to "give nature a helping hand," and to append one's own indelible trademark to one's body. After all, does each and *every* designer not choose his or her own label? Why then, should a woman not be allowed to hit the spot with her own design?

Chapter XVIII

Freckles

Freckles doubtless deserve the name given to them in the mid-eighteenth century — as poetic as it is wise — of "ephelides" (from the Greek "epi," meaning "because of," and "helios," "sun").

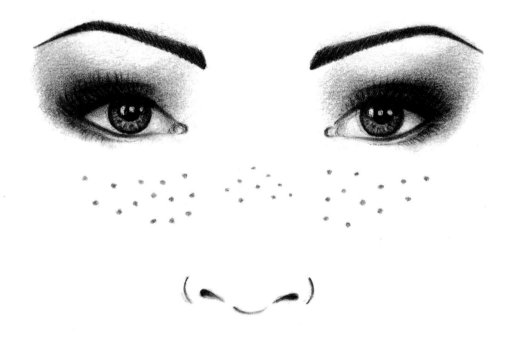

Freckles give their owners a youthful and impish look. They are associated with sound health, nature, and sun. They are therefore much sought after and can be achieved with the help of permanent makeup. However, tattooed freckles can only be applied to certain "woody" skins. These are skin tones where freckles can appear naturally. A brown or olive complexion does not usually have these characteristics and freckles would look unnatural.

The key words, when it comes to drawing freckles, are "discretion and delicacy." They are tiny and orangy-yellow to light golden brown in color. The skin in the "W"-shaped area, straddling the nose where they are drawn, is very vascular. This can lead to the tattoo becoming enlarged.

The shape and regularity of each of these tiny freckles should vary greatly. It is important that this small "deception" should remain undetected.

If we are to believe the word, naturally occurring ephelides appear "because of the sun." In reality, they already exist, but they only appear *in* the sun. This is not the case when freckles are created through permanent makeup. Exposure to the sun is more likely to make them fade as the face acquires a tan. It is important to know this in advance so that you are prepared. The contrast between the tan and these freckles will be less marked when you go out in the sun. But after all, the aim of "ephelides" created in this way is to make your life easier, and does their beauty not "make up" for all the hours you cannot spend in the sun?

Chapter XIX
Rouge/Blusher

Her noble modesty brought color to her cheeks…
—Jean Racine, *Phaedra*, Act II, Sc 5

Morning was always kind to her.
On her cheeks she wore her rosy hues.
—Colette, *La Maison de Claudine*

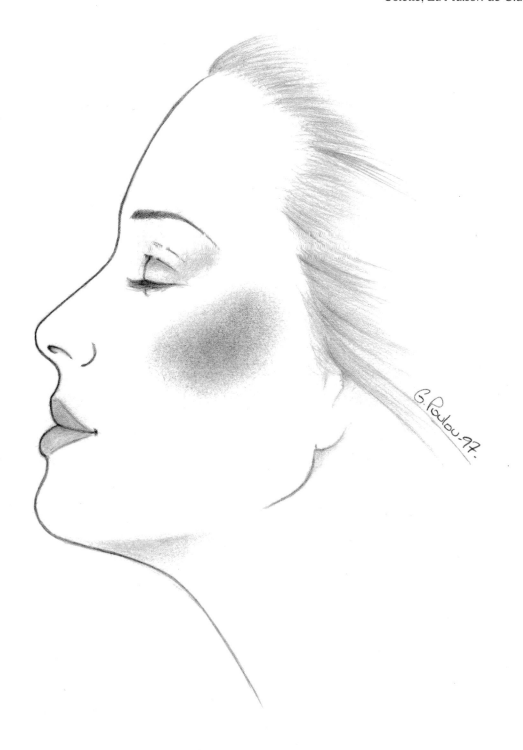

I like to be reminded, by the diaphanous cloud skillfully abandoned on your cheeks, of the tempests and environments that bring color to them: fresh air, feelings, enthusiasm, joy. It is a positive coloration (the blush of shame, on the other hand, appears on the brow, not the cheeks...).

There are two distinct, different ways to make up the cheeks and/or cheekbones:

✓ *"molding" blush*: where we "sculpt" the face to produce, through the use of dark casts (brown, gold, or copper tones), more contoured cheeks and/or cheekbones.

✓ *"healthy glow" blush*: where we highlight with pink and bring color to the cheeks and/or cheekbones (and sometimes a touch of color to the chin).

In permanent makeup, we only apply the "healthy glow" blush[1], for it is the only one really worthy of the name.

When the brown tones are introduced "straight into the skin," as they fade or alter with the passing of time, they can often give the cheeks an unhealthy glow (which is not the case when the eyebrows fade). Moreover, as our tan changes several times a year, tattooed brown blusher will look too pale on a suntanned face and too dark on a pale face (this can look particularly unattractive). Clients who want *permanent makeup* on their cheeks, are strongly advised to opt for the "healthy glow blush" and to leave the "molding blush" to *cosmetic makeup*.

To obtain a *lighter and more transparent* effect, we use a very diluted rosy-red (75% distilled water to 25% pigment), so that the application has less "volume." The opposite effect will be obtained if you try to lighten the blusher with *white*, as this will make the colors drab and opaque[2].

In permanent makeup, really natural looking blusher (along with freckles) is one of the most difficult effects to achieve. For we do not draw a line but deposit a *cloud* that has to blend lightly, subtly, and gradually with the skin tone. It is crucial, therefore, that the person who applies it has been well trained in this particular technique. It is not enough to have been trained in the application of lip contour, eyebrows, or eyeliner.

Only go ahead with blusher if you feel confident you will be able to happily turn the other cheek!

> *Thy cheeks shew*
> *through their veil rosy*
> *as a halved pomegranate.*
> —Song of Songs, IV, 3

[1]"Blush" comes from the word "Blood"
[2]White is not a color that has volume; see chapter entitled: "Colors"

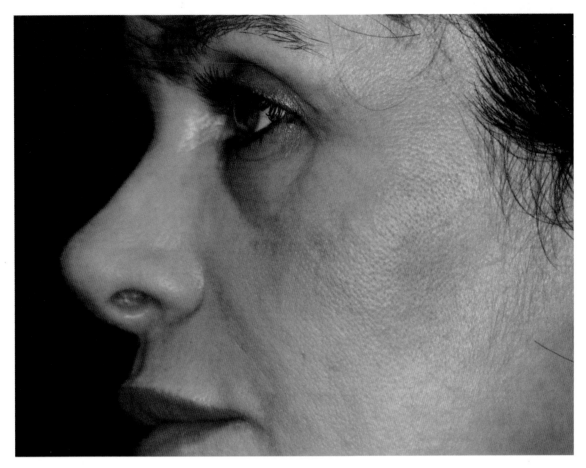

Rouge/Blusher.

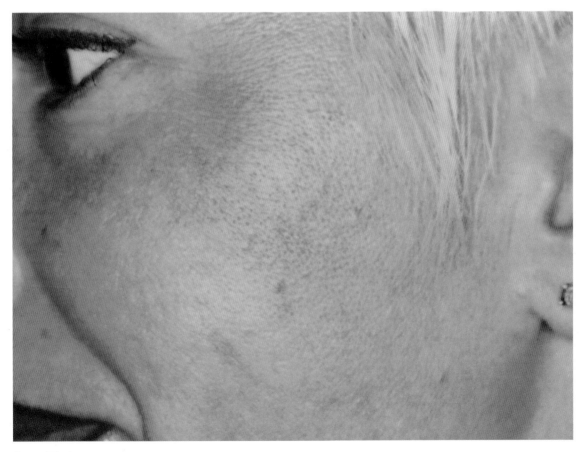

Rouge/Blusher.

Chapter XX

Paramedical Applications

*On a face a defect of the soul cannot be corrected
but a defect of the face, if it is corrected,
can correct a soul.*
—Jean Cocteau

Many men and women are disfigured as a result of accidents, illness, birth defects, and even surgery. These defects are permanent. Cosmetic makeup is only a temporary solution. So, what can be done?

When your self-image and self-confidence have been damaged, reconstructive dermagraphics can help restore your zest for life.

When a person has had an operation to correct *a birth defect* (a classic example is the cleft-lip), scarring is inevitable. It is the same when someone undergoes surgery as a result of an *accident* (e.g. facial injuries sustained in a car crash) or *illness* (operation for breast cancer). Certain types of *cosmetic surgery* can also leave scars (e.g. breast reductions and facelifts). No blame can be attached to the surgeon; some scars are just simply inevitable and we all "scar" differently.

Reconstructive dermagraphics can sometimes be the "final touch" to surgery.

The cleft-lip

The cleft-lip is a congenital disorder. During fetal development the palate area fails to close completely and one or two fissures remain. Sometimes it only affects the upper lip, at other times it affects the nose, resulting in differently shaped nostrils. Corrective surgery is done early in infancy.

When this type of corrective surgery deforms the shape of the mouth, reconstructive dermapigmentation can often produce some excellent results. We redraw the "Cupid's bow," which is the area usually affected. Lip contour gives the mouth a more regular shape and the pigmentation of the actual lips, within the line, completes the illusion of an absolutely normal mouth.

The reconstitution of the lips through reconstructive dermapigmentation dates from 1858 (Dr Schuh in Vienna)[1].

Scalp

Dermagraphics is not recommended as a solution to the essentially male, age-related problem of gradual (or galloping) hair loss. It would need to be applied regularly in a desperate and futile race against the inevitable onset of baldness. Can you picture the somewhat unattractive end result? The only viable proposition for this problem is a hair transplant, which usually consists of carrying out a series of micrografts in order to shrink the bald areas. This often entails long-term treatment and a shading-off, by means of permanent makeup, of the bare patches on the scalp or between the grafts. In this situation, permanent makeup can offer an interesting short-term, illusory solution.

There is no surgical solution to the more uncommon condition of female baldness since the whole of the scalp is affected (there are no bald areas, just general thinning of hair). Permanent makeup can therefore offer a solution.

When the problem is the result of an accident — burns or an operation that leaves bald areas on the scalp — it is possible to tattoo individual hairs, thereby creating an illusion of hair.

Beard, moustache

Lack of hair growth in these areas is frequently due to scarring, the result of an accident or an operation to correct a cleft-lip.

✓ **In an area that is shaved** (such as the chin or cheeks), dots are tattooed to imitate stubble. For a more natural look, we choose a color that is one tone lighter than the natural facial hair.

✓ **In the beard or moustache**, the procedure is the same as for the scalp. We use a color that matches the root.

Pubic hair

This is done to camouflage a scar on the pubis following an operation such as a caesarian. If the operation has shortened the distance between the edge of the pubis and the navel, we are careful to ensure that the dermapigmentation does not accentuate the optical illusion.

Breast areolas

✓ **To camouflage a periareolary scar**: The inverted T-shaped (or "anchor") scar that results from breast reduction due to mammary hypertrophy or ptosis (sagging) fades with time. But the circular or serrated ones, left around the areola when round block reduction is carried out, can be visually embarrassing. By stimulating the areola color the scar is brought into the areola.

✓ **To recreate an areola with "3-dimensional" nipple**: the lack of an areola arises from a complete or partial mastectomy due to the presence of cancer. Dermagraphics is particularly welcomed since the procedure does not entail the "patient" having to be admitted to hospital, being administered an anesthetic, or needing to take time off work.

✓ **Recoloration of a grafted areola**: when a surgeon undertakes the reconstruction of an areola and nipple, it can be too pale or unnatural looking.

✓ **Not involving surgery**: some people (women and men) do not like having areolas that are too small, too pale, or badly defined.

Scar therapy

Camouflaging scars "straight into the skin" is one of the most difficult procedures to undertake. Why? Because just as with fingerprints there are as many skin tones as there are individuals on the planet.

Whereas in other forms of tattooing and permanent makeup we select a color that *stands out* from the skin, in this instance we have to find the color *closest* to the natural skin tone.

We must therefore identify the skin color and its underlying tone (see Chapter IX, "Why and How to Identify Skin Tone). This could be blue, green, red, yellow, copper, etc.

Moreover, while the color of the procedure will not change, skin color can vary according to whether the person is hot or cold, healthy or ill, tanned or not (sun, tanning beds, self-tanning lotions, etc.).

First we draw the missing areola to look as much like the other as far as position and shape are concerned.

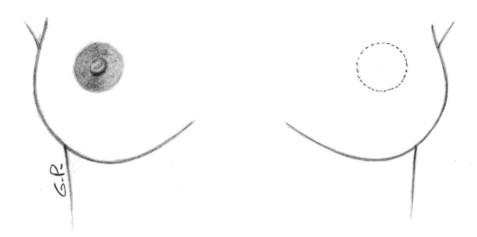

Then we tattoo the areola, reproducing any variation of color present on the other breast, so that the effect is as natural as possible.

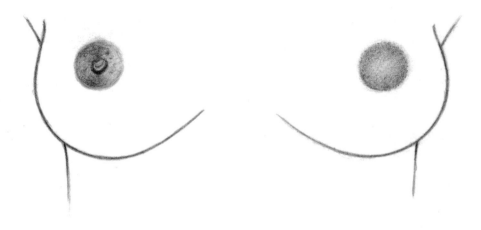

Finally, we do the edge of the nipple, making it darker in color than the areola, so that it appears to stand out. The skill lies in making the whole look three-dimensional.

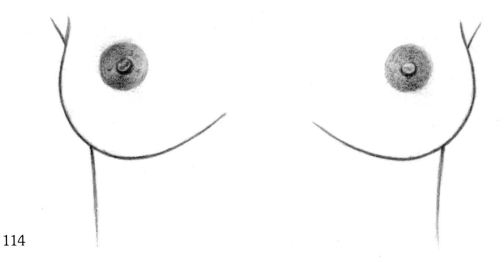

The best results are obtained when the scar is *lighter* than the surrounding area. Whilst we can never achieve perfection (for the above mentioned reasons), there is a distinct improvement.

If the scar is darker[2], the lighter camouflage is not always very satisfactory: it can appear "chalky" and look as though it is "floating" above the skin.

It is also easier when the scar is flat. With depressed or bulging scars, the skin does not catch the light in the same way, with the result that the pigmentation will not always turn out as expected.

Vitiligo and other forms of depigmentation

Vitiligo is a chronic form of depigmentation. It affects around 0.5% of the population and the cause is unknown[3]. It can cover the whole body or only a small area. Contrary to what is generally believed, it does not only affect dark-skinned people. It is frequently found on the face, around the eyes, nostrils, mouth, and on the hands. It can work its way towards the eyebrows and into the scalp and can result in loss of hair pigment.

Vitiligo is unpredictable. Initially, it might be no more than a slight nuisance. But it can spread gradually over a period of several years. It can suddenly manifest itself following a period of stress or severe sunburn. It arises from the destruction of the melanocytes. Biopsies carried out on these white areas have revealed a loss of melanocytes.

The tattooing of vitiligo is an extremely delicate procedure. It is, in fact, so unreliable that many practitioners refuse to do it. It would appear that the stress caused by the procedure itself can cause the condition to spread.

In the case of vitiligo, it is absolutely essential to know, before proceeding, how the white areas have grown. Have they increased in size, are they spreading to the arms or legs? Only if the condition has remained stable over a three-year period should treatment even be considered.

Before opting for tattooing, it is advisable to follow a course of PUVA[5] treatment or to use a camouflaging makeup[4]. This has proved most effective in approximately 60% of cases (but less effective in such areas as the mouth, face, hands, and feet).

By *decreasing the contrast* between the "normal" area and the depigmented area, dermapigmentation can make vitiligo less noticeable.

✓ **The depigmented area**: We "stipple" the area in much the same way that a photographer touches up a photograph. The operation requires a lot of patience and several sessions. We begin with light dots and then progressively darker dots, until we have produced the right tone. We use *several* flesh-colored tones, for if we were to limit ourselves to one or two, the final effect would not look natural enough.

The technique can in fact be used to pigment scars and other areas of depigmentation. It must be understood however that its application is for permanent achromia and dyschromia[6] only, and not for temporary conditions (if in doubt, consult your doctor).

[1]Zwerling, Walker, Goldstein, *Micropigmentation, State of the Art*, USA, p. 14; C. Bruno, *Tatoués, qui êtes-vous?* Paris 1970, p. 153.

[2]See Chapter XI on "Hyperpigmentation."

[3]This and other data on vitiligo has been taken from Zwerling, Walker, Goldstein, *Micropigmentation, State of the Art*, USA, 1993, p. 176 ff.

[4]Like Covermark™

[5]Psoralen - ultraviolet "A" Light.

[6]Achromia = absence of color. Dyschromia = difference of color.

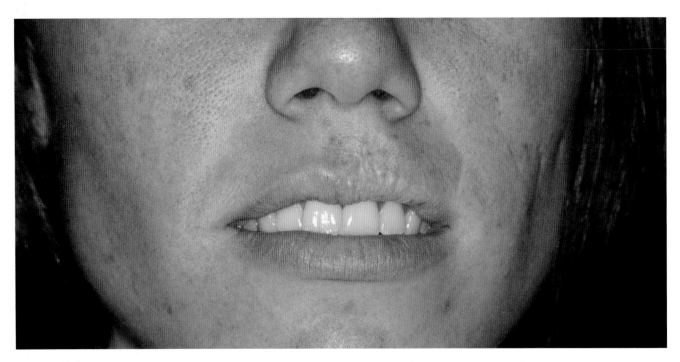

Before.

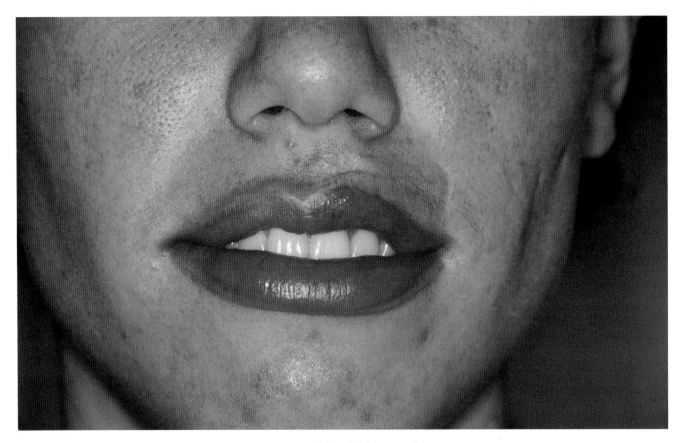

Immediately after procedure. *Courtesy of Kristanne Matzek / American Institute.*

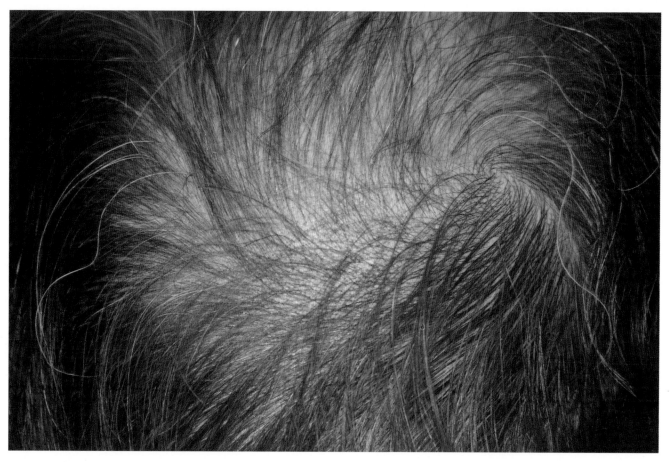

After receiving two hair transplantations…

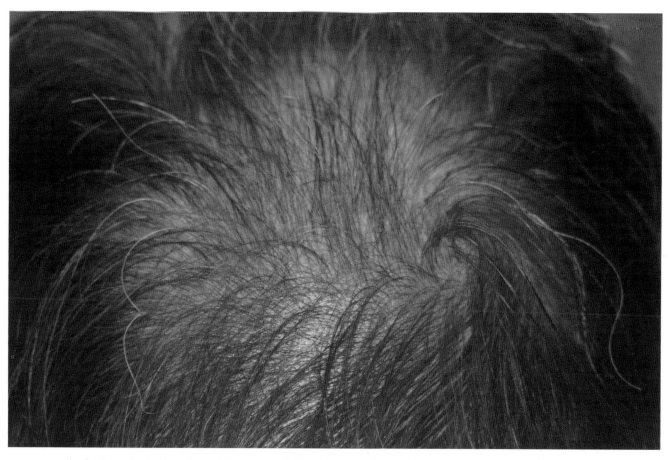

…the final touch of micropigmentation completed to this patient's satisfaction.

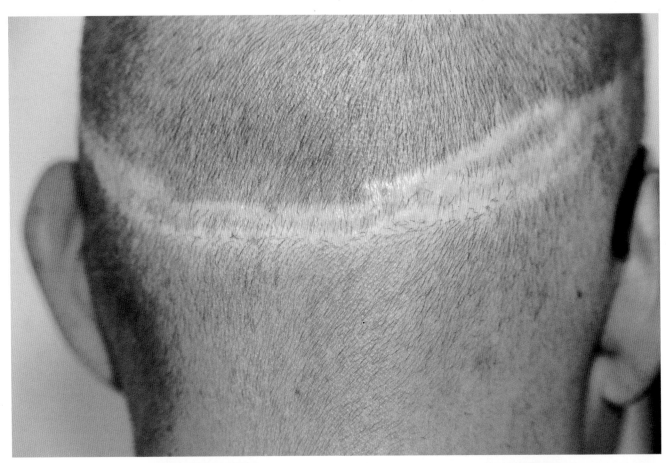

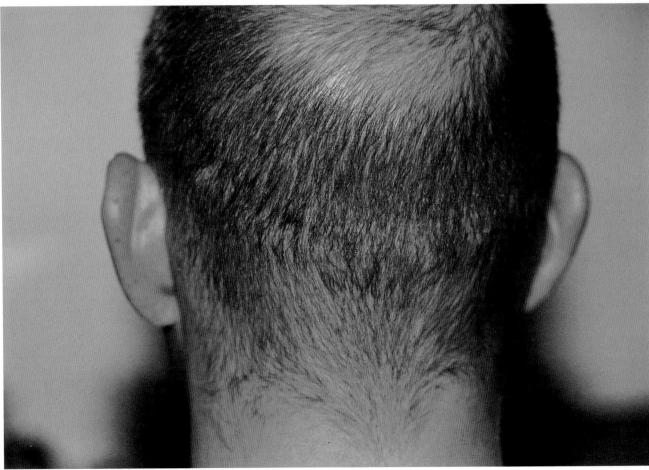

Hair transplant donor site scar, camouflaged with both skin tone repigmentation and tattooed hairstrokes.
Courtesy of Jeffery Lyle Segal (Chicago, IL and Beverly Hills, CA).

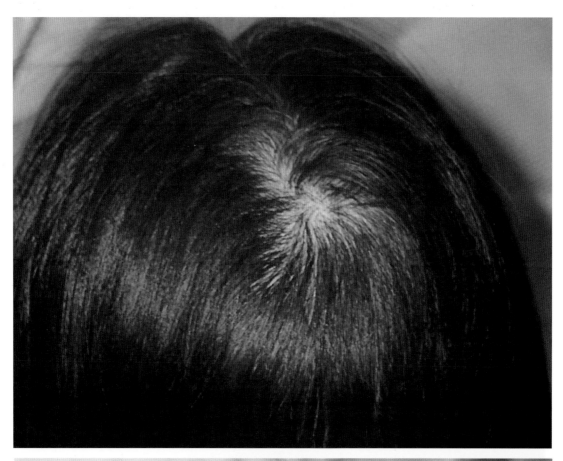

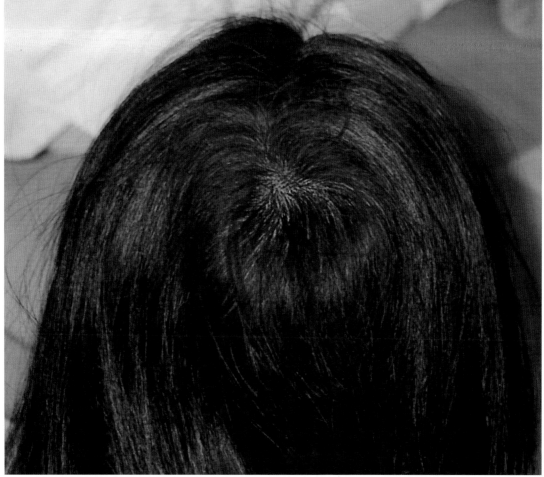

Camouflaging thin hair on crown. *Courtesy of Kristanne Matzek / American Institute.*

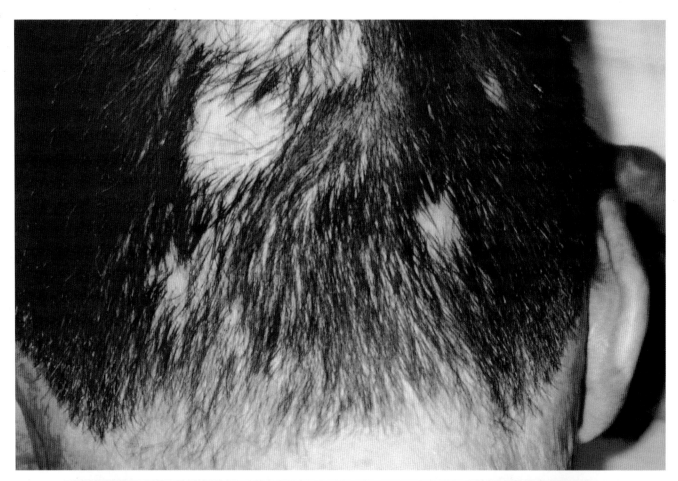

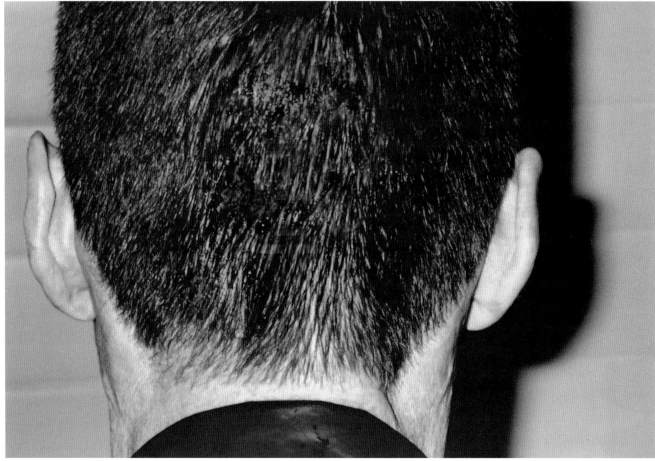

Permanent cosmetic hair simulation. *Courtesy of Dominique Bossavy.*

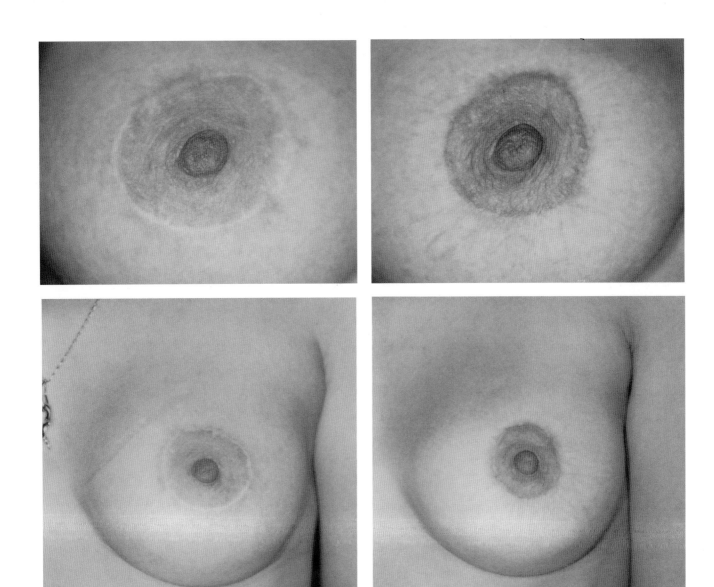

Camouflaging a periareolary scar after breast augmentation.

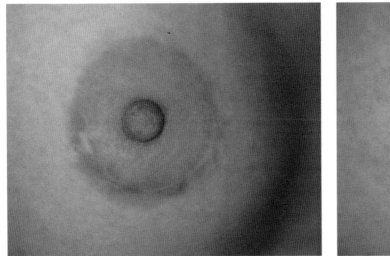

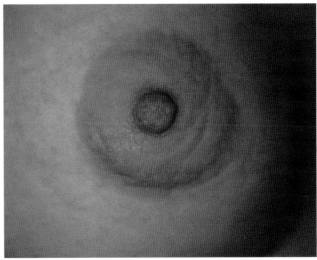

Camouflaging small scars after breast augmentation.

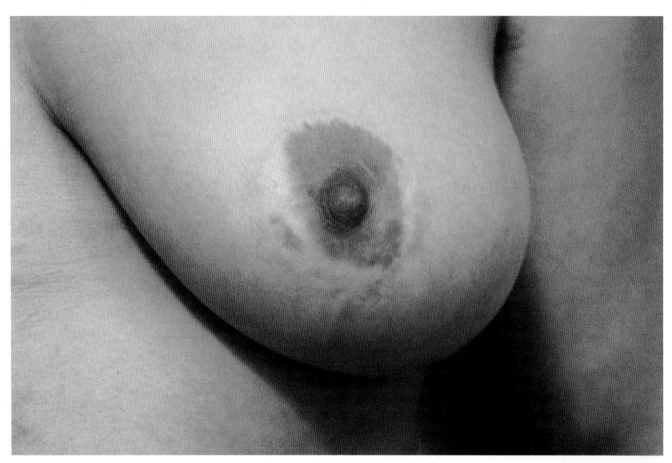

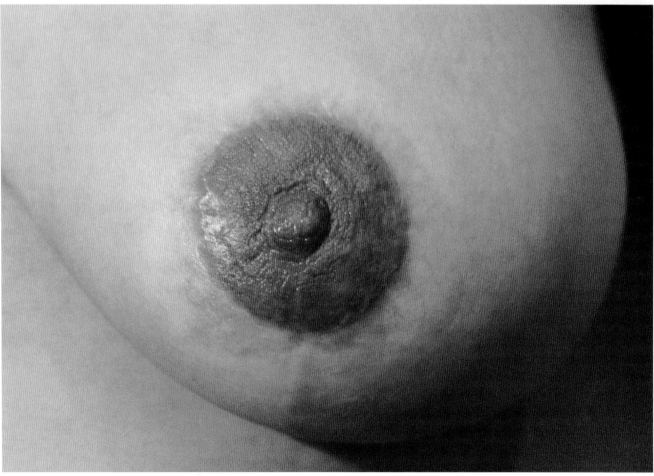

Scar camouflage after breast reduction.

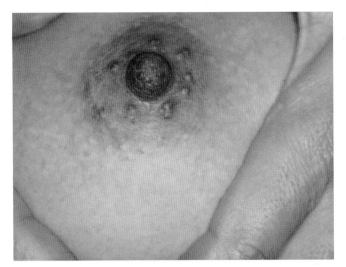
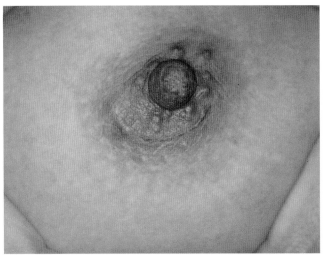

Camouflaging small scars after breast augmentation.

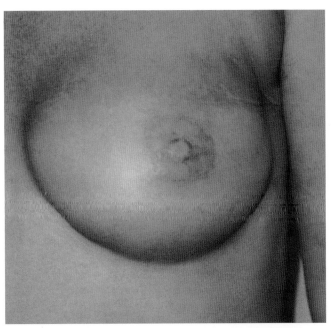
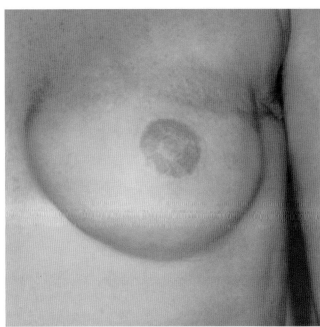

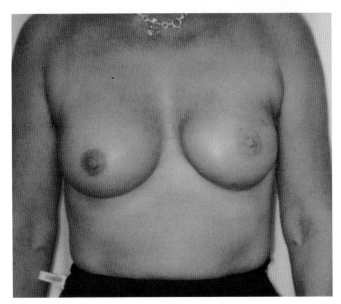
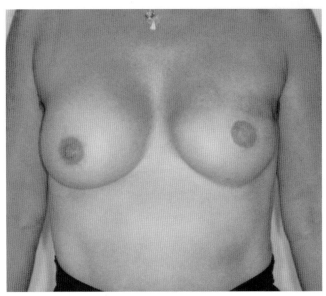

Pigmentation of the areola following mastectomy and breast reconstruction.

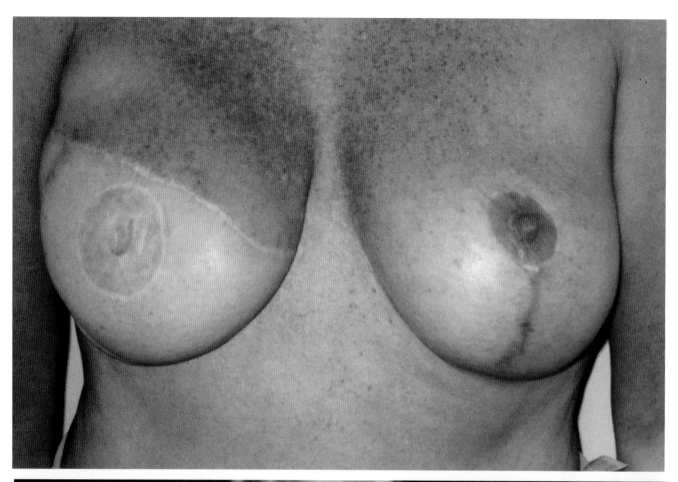

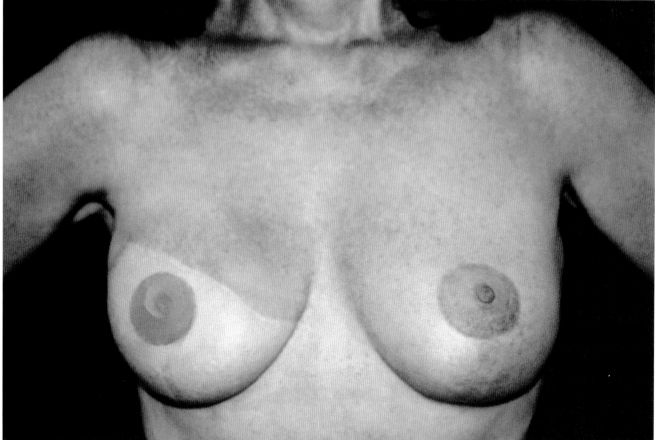

Asymmetry correction in post mastectomy patient. Enlargement of the left areola and pigmentation of the right areola. *Courtesy of Dominique Bossavy.*

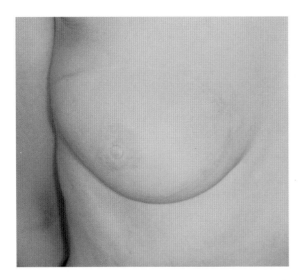
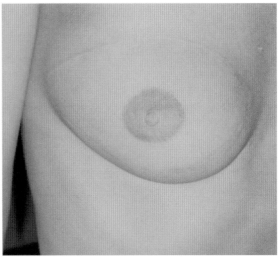

Pigmentation of the grafted areola after mastectomy with breast reconstruction.

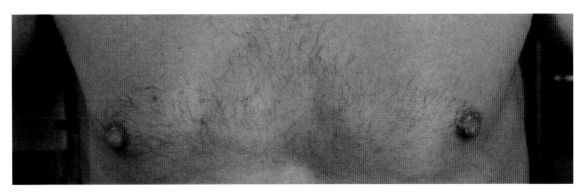

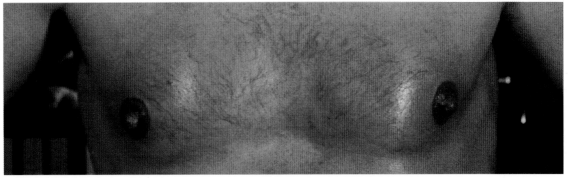

Enlarging areolas for a man adds symmetry to the chest.

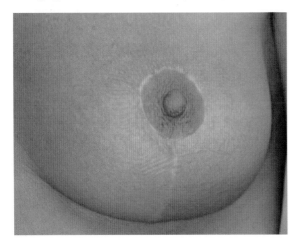
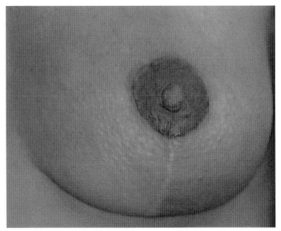

Scar camouflage after breast reduction.

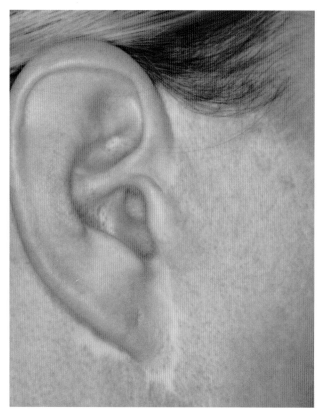
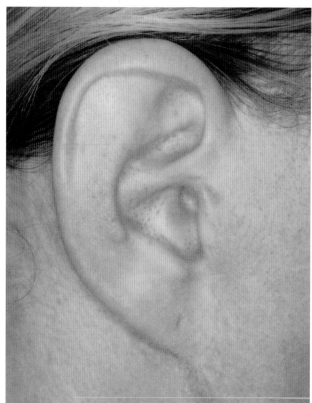

Camouflaging scar after face lift.

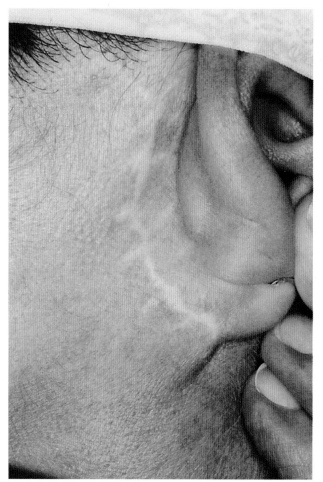
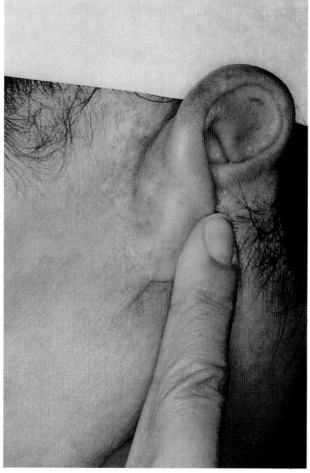

Pigmentation of scar after facelift. *Courtesy of Danny Attali, Paris.*

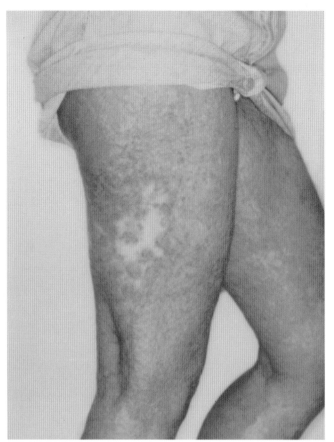
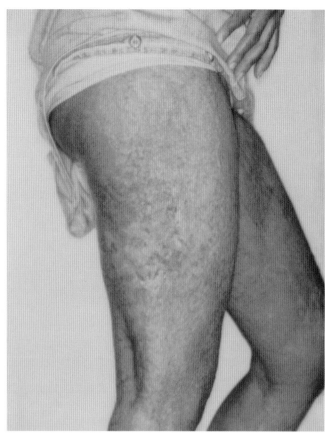
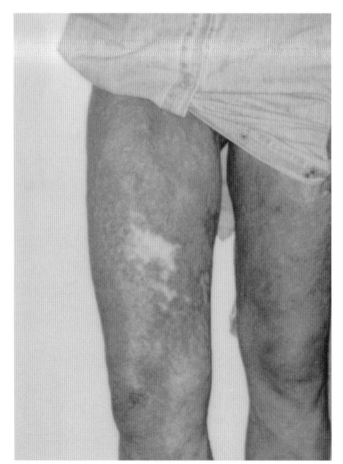
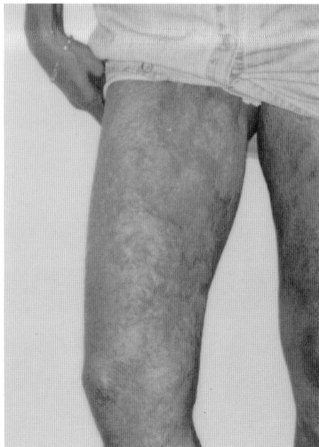

Camouflaging grafted skin after burns.

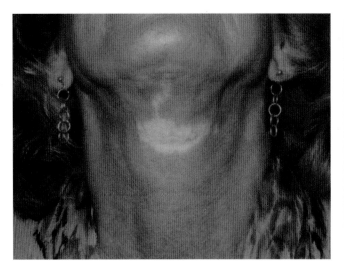
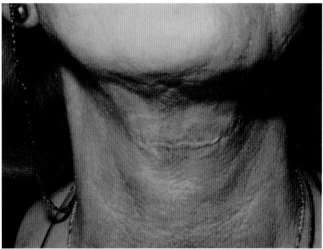

Post procedure camouflaging vitiligo. *Courtesy of Bonnie Ripper.*

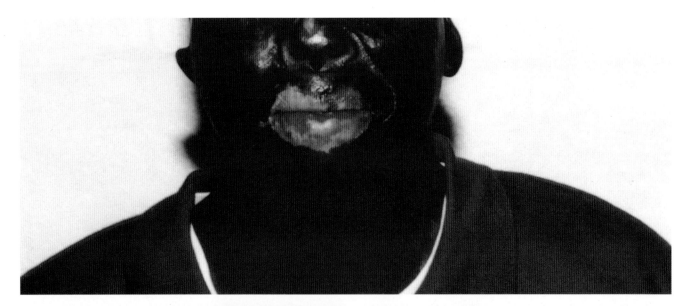

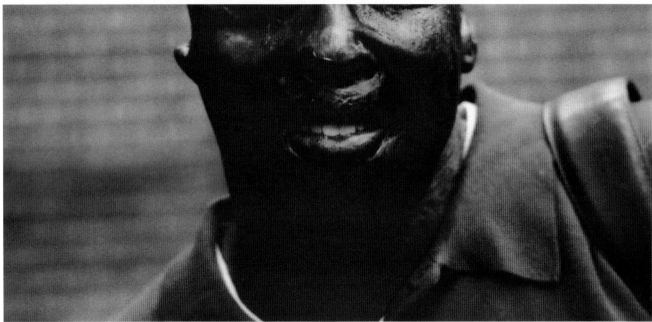

Camouflage of hypopigmentation caused by vitiligo. *Courtesy of Dominique Bossavy.*

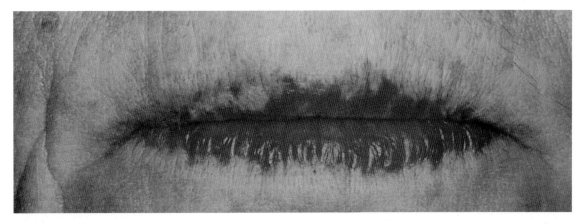

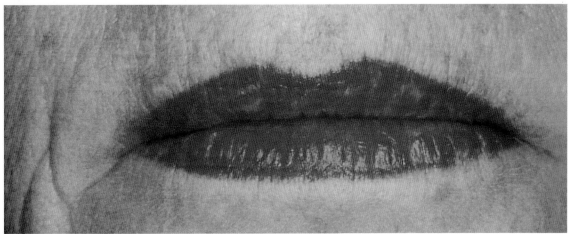

Camouflage of hypopigmentation caused by vitiligo. *Courtesy of Danny Attali, Paris.*

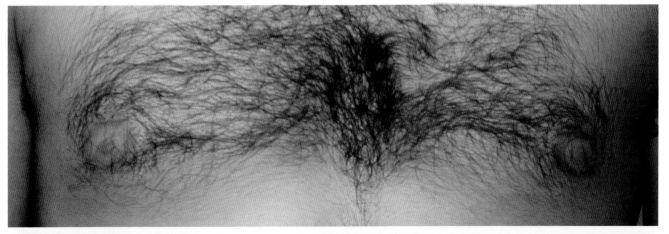

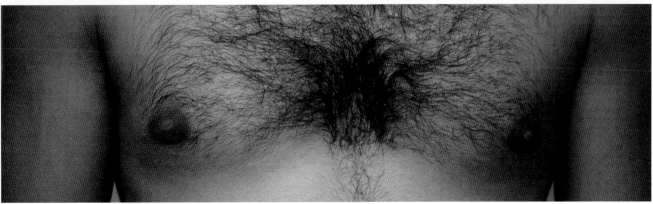

Camouflaging vitiligo of the areolas.

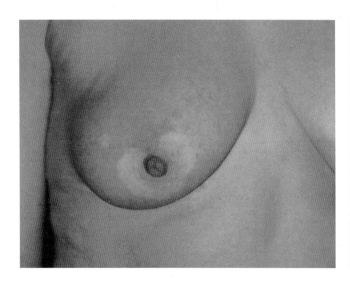
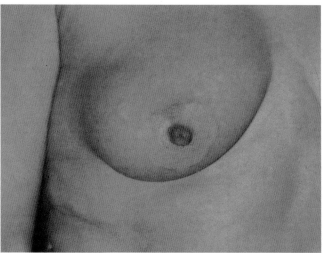

Camouflaging vitiligo around the nipple after one procedure. A second procedure will be necessary to achieve perfect matching with skin color.

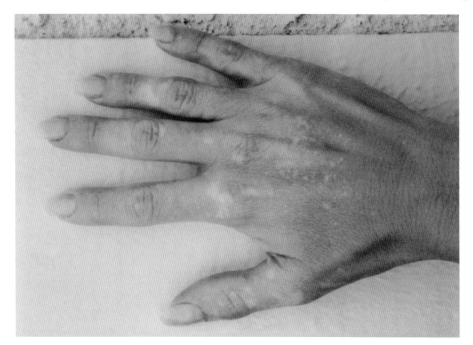

Camouflaging vitiligo.
Courtesy of Kristanne Matzek.

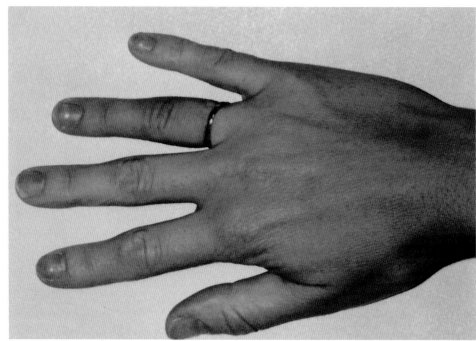

130

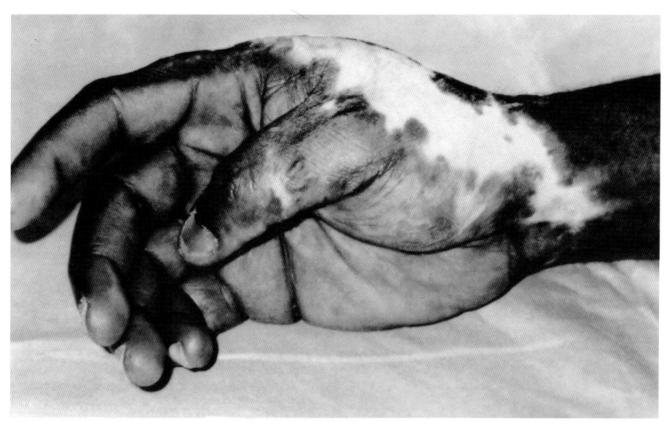

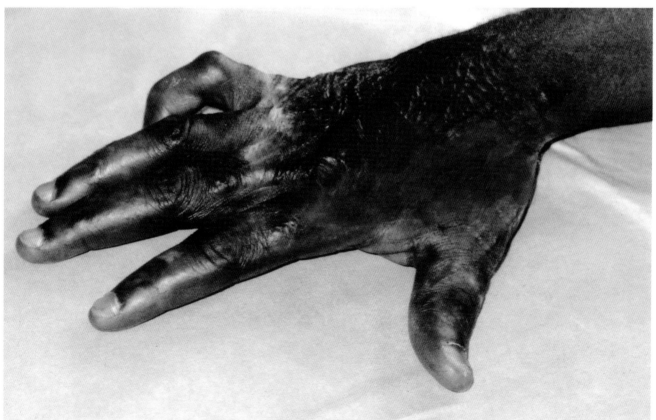

Camouflaging vitiligo. *Courtesy of Dominique Bossavy.*

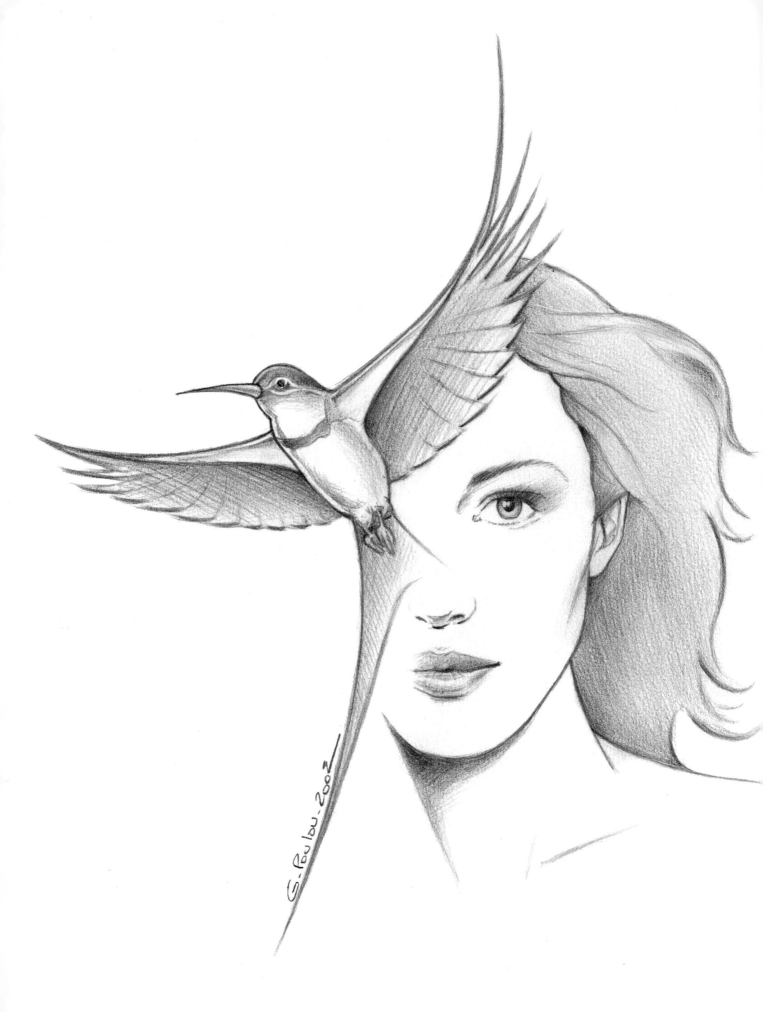

Chapter XXI
Beyond the Scar

By Anne-Dominique Bossavy[1], Los Angeles, California

Cosmetic and Reconstructive Micropigmentation
Honored member, Phoenix Deutschland for burn survivors
Award of Excellence of the AAM[2], 2002

Like a soul bruised by cruel destiny,
Like a heart scratched by the thorn of experience,
You've survived by clinging to the roots of life.
Your vulnerability became strength,
Your despair became hope,
Your fear turned into courage,
Your knowledge became wisdom,
Your self-esteem is beauty,
And alike a cocoon, YOU become a butterfly.
—A.D.B

As a micropigmentation practitioner with many years of experience, specializing in camouflage application, I've seen how people with burns manage to cope and adjust to the results of their injuries. Although some people will say that one who hasn't suffered a burn injury cannot fundamentally understand the experience of dealing with burn disfigurement, I've dealt with hundreds of people who have suffered the devastation of burns, and have assisted and witnessed many of them in their efforts to live a normal life.

The experience of living with burn disfigurement and coping with the corresponding physical and emotional suffering, the brutal change in appearance, and the loss of identity can be an overwhelming experience. But often these trying circumstances produce the most successful, productive, and generous human beings I have ever met.

The alteration in one's life can ultimately be a positive one. Some individuals who accept their condition with remarkable wisdom and strength can inspire all who are around them with their humor and vitality. However, in most cases, the road to gaining back self-confidence, self-esteem, and self-acceptance is a long one.

Camouflage micropigmentation treatment has proven very helpful for patients wishing to minimize the emotional problems directly linked to their appearance in a more "permanent" way.

Patients who have camouflage micropigmentation procedures applied do not consider it a luxury, as is the case with purely cosmetic applications (such as lip liner, eyeliner, or eyebrow enhancement), but rather a necessity to improve their appearance and self-image. They find it undeniably valuable in restoring emotional balance in their lives, offering them new options and new hope to face the world more comfortably.

The consultation

In my practice I am often brought face to face with patients whose features are so distorted that in some cases I can hardly recognize them as human beings. I make it my priority to make this patient feel comfortable. Doing otherwise would rob the patient of dignity. Being professional doesn't mean being impersonal. The tremendous anxiety for the future, the repulsion at a reconstructed face, and rejection from the public make the burn survivor patient very sensitive. In this regard, I find it extremely important not to leave the disfigured patient seated in a waiting room full of other patients who might stare.

Life circumstance has damaged the outside but these individuals are still the same on the inside. I would like to emphasize that patients suffering disfigurement are more than survivors — we must consider them heroes. Although the practitioner must recognize this patient's vulnerability, it is equally important to recognize and honor their courage, for they have made it through so much.

"The eyes are the window of the soul"

When meeting with a severely disfigured person, it is best if the practitioner genuinely smiles and looks into their eyes, to meet the person on the inside. A practitioner should not look directly at the disfigurement and appear sad, appalled, or curious. By holding the patient's hands, by showing that they are not repulsed by the patient's appearance, the practitioner will make the patient feel at ease.

Designing the treatment

Before undertaking a camouflage micropigmentation procedure, the practitioner must design and develop in concert with the patient a plan of treatment that provides the patient with different aesthetic options. It is for the patient to choose the suggestion that feels most comfortable and attractive, and that best camouflages the defects. In order to avoid false expectations that would have devastating effects on the patient's emotional and psychological well-being, the practitioner must assist the patient to fully understand the possibilities and limitations of camouflage micropigmentation by clearly explaining to him or her what can be achieved as well as what cannot be achieved.

To insure full satisfaction, it is mandatory for patients to understand and accept that camouflage micropigmentation will improve their appearance but rarely will this procedure bring them back to the way they were before the accident.

Communication

Clear communication between the patient and practitioner is the key to successful treatment. It involves allowing the patient to express fear and dislike freely in a space where what he or she says will not be judged or analyzed.

Listening

By genuinely listening, the practitioner encourages the patient to share valuable information. This will assist the practitioner in developing a plan of treatment that will best resolve the patient issues.

During this very first phase of the treatment, it is important for the patient to feel safe in confiding and expressing his psychological and emotional concerns to the practitioner. On the other end, the words spoken by the practitioner must reflect genuine caring and a commitment to assist.

The practitioner must keep in mind that not all patients will accept the change easily. On the contrary, it is quite normal for the patient to resist and fear the change. Life is forever altered for this patient who has to adjust to the stranger now seen in the mirror. It will take time to adjust to the new change. It is the responsibility of the practitioner to guide the patient in visualizing the self more realistically, thus insuring full satisfaction with the final results.

The treatment

Performing camouflage micropigmentation to assist severely disfigured people will sometimes bring the biggest challenges as well as the greatest rewards. Facial reconstruction, in some cases, can be a long process that often requires multiple complex corrective surgeries. For this reason, it is best for the patient to seek a micropigmentation specialist who will work in concert with the surgeon caring for the patient's reconstructive surgeries.

The ultimate solution is the combination of the fine reconstructive work of the surgeon — who often has reconstructed an entire face — and the final touch of the micropigmentation specialists.

Whether micropigmentation specialists are providing corrective camouflage micropigmentation, treatments in a salon, in a doctor's office, or in a hospital, they must be knowledgeable and experienced in determining how to conduct a treatment that will truly help these patients and make a difference in their lives physically, and most importantly, emotionally.

When performing camouflage micropigmentation, my primary concern is to correct skin color defects, asymmetry problems, and create the illusion of smoother skin. This re-establishes a well-defined and balanced face, recreating as normal an appearance as scientifically and artistically possible. I make it my goal to help these patients re-enter and blend into mainstream society, thus giving them back their self-image, self-esteem, and social acceptance — qualities that had been taken away from them by their traumatic condition.

Extreme precision is needed. For the burn survivor the smallest imperfection can make a world of difference in the way a person feels about himself.

"Something is not better then nothing..."

When chosen and trusted to make a difference, the practitioner must make sure it will be a good one. I like to think of my patients as if they were extremely valuable pieces of art that life had damaged, and my role is to restore them. I make certain they leave my office feeling armed with the best camouflage micropigmentation possible, in order to face and find a place in society.

Camouflage micropigmentation not only affects the altered appearance, but also the psychological, social, and emotional well being. The "boost" in self-esteem, reflecting from the restored picture, is undeniable.

[1]www.europeanacademy.org
[2]American Academy of Micropigmentation

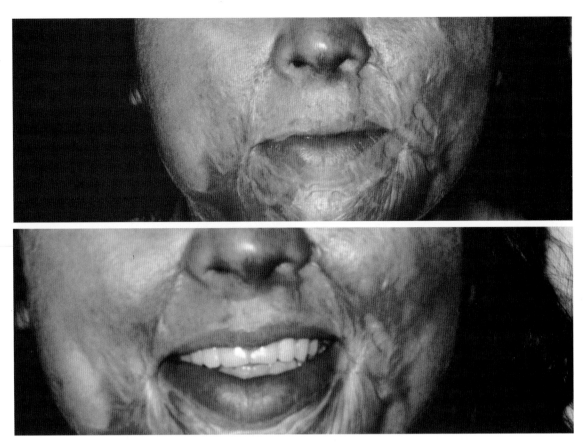

Full lips. *Courtesy of Dominique Bossavy.*

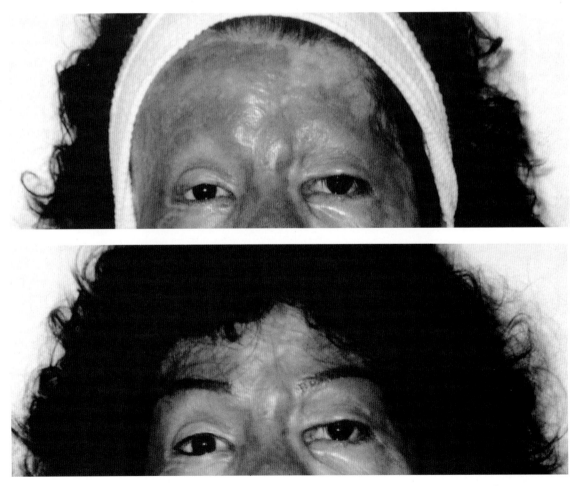

Eyebrows and eyeliner on the right eye creating balance with the left eye. *Courtesy of Dominique Bossavy.*

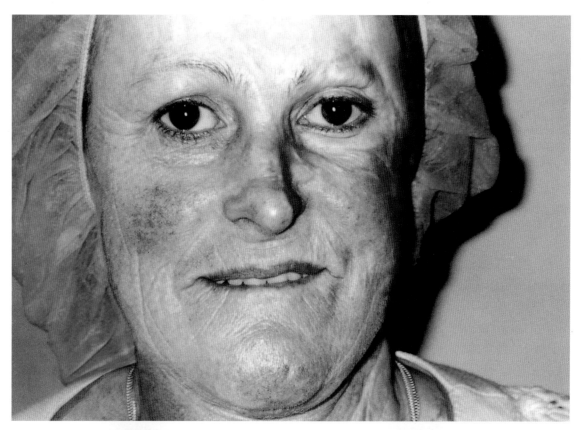

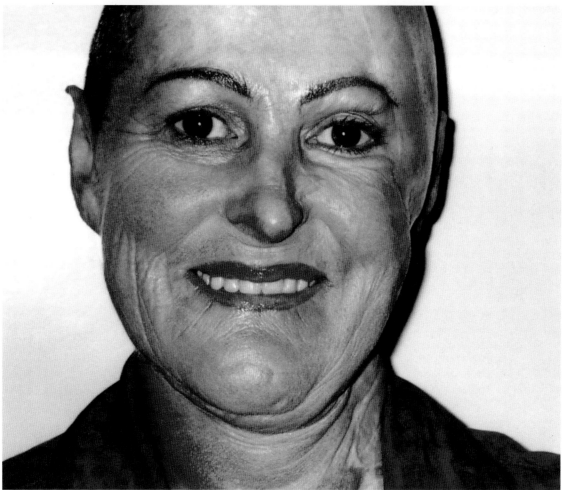

Eyebrows, full lips, and liner, immediately after procedure, restoring the facial expression.
Courtesy of Dominique Bossavy.

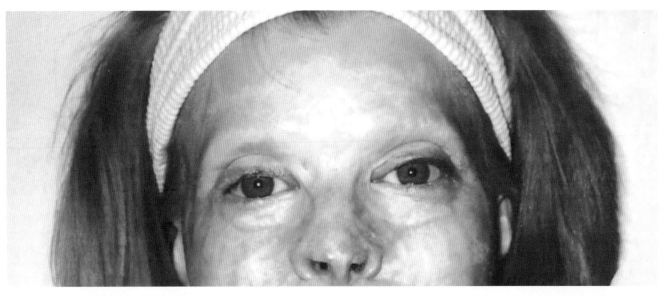

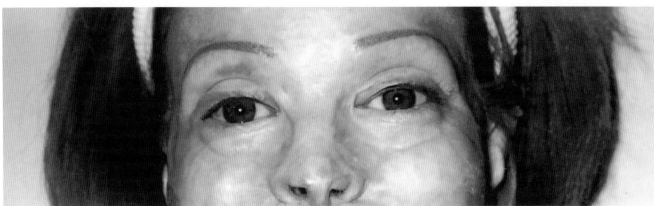

Eyebrows and eyeliner immediately after procedure. *Courtesy of Dominique Bossavy.*

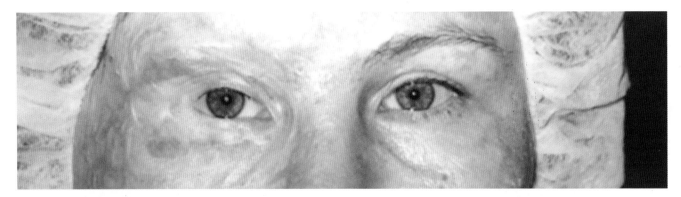

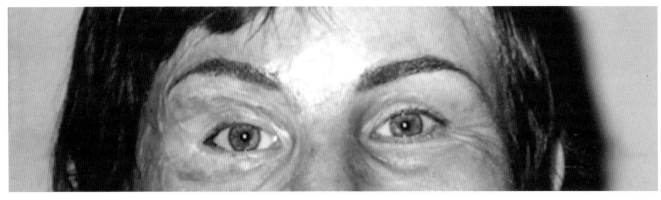

Eyebrows and pigmentation of the right eyeliner to recreate balance with left side, just after procedure. *Courtesy of Dominique Bossavy.*

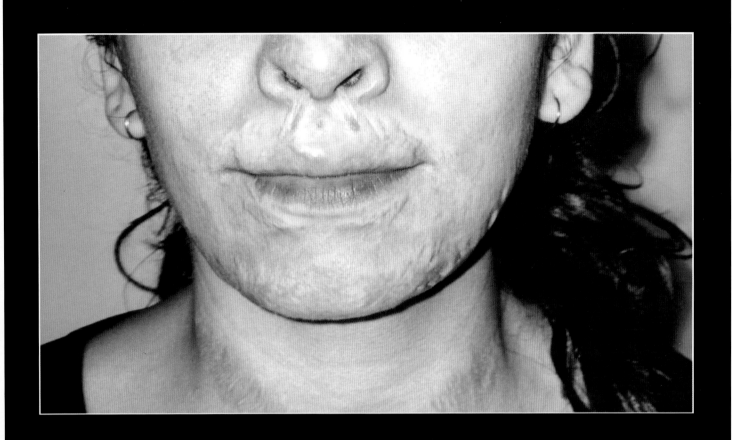

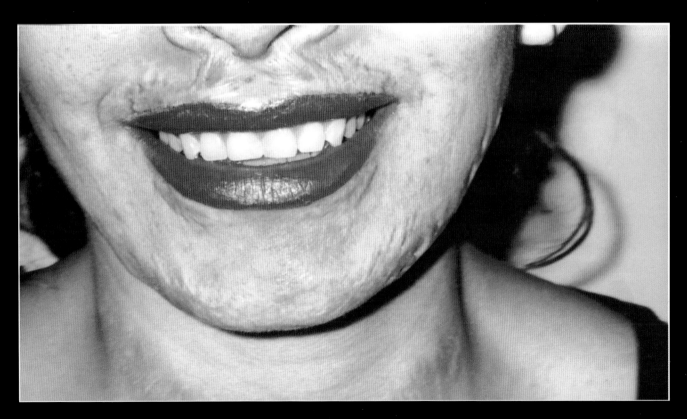

Multritrepanic collagen actuation, or scar releasing (*see* Chapters XX and XXII), and pigmentation of the full lipcolor just after. *Courtesy of Dominique Bossavy.*

Chapter XXII
Multitrepannic[1] Collagen Actuation (MCA)

MCA is a new method of dermapigmentation, first developed by Dr. Adrianna Schreibner, a laser specialist[2]. MCA utilizes a "dry needle" technique (i.e. containing no pigment) in order to:

✓ soften and flatten scars
✓ stimulate the natural recoloration of a scar that is white
✓ stimulate natural recoloration in small areas of vitiligo
✓ improve the appearance of wrinkles

To soften and flatten scars[3]

A single needle stipples the skin by puncturing it. The intensity and direction of the needle's movement must be exact so that any damage to the surrounding healthy tissue is kept to a minimum. A circular, backward, or forward movement can, on the other hand, cause a build-up of collagen, and therefore worsen the scar. When such scars are found on the eyebrows or lips, for example, it is strongly recommended to undergo this treatment and then await the result *before* going ahead with permanent makeup.

To stimulate the natural recoloration of a scar that is white

While the laser is especially useful when it comes to *removing colorations* of the skin (tattoos, strawberry birthmarks, other birth marks, age spots, hyperpigmenation, etc.), Dr. Schreibner also worked on hypopigmented (lack of color) areas of the skin, with the aim of getting them to *recolor* themselves naturally.

In order to understand this process fully, it should be noted that the function of the *epidermis* is to form a barrier against lesions and the action of toxic agents. It protects the body and the dermis, the innermost layer of the skin. As well as other factors, the epidermis contains *melanocytes*, pigment-producing cells (tanning) that shield us from the harmful effects of the sun.

The *dermis* is composed of naturally produced collagen, which is indispensable to the *scarring mechanism*. It has been found, through examining a scar, that a trauma suffered by the skin stimulates the production of collagen, which then crosses the layers of the skin to replace the epidermis. Because the dermis contains no melanocytes (they occur in the epidermis), the scar is hypopigmented (lacking in color). For color to re-occur naturally in this area, it is necessary to restore melanocytes to the scar tissue so that they can produce pigments.

By exposing scar tissue to a laser beam, Dr. Schreibner observed on more than one occasion that while the former was reacting to this "minor trauma," collagen was being "re-instated." However, no superfluous collagen formed. On the contrary, it had disappeared, in much the same way that the color of a tattoo is dispersed when subjected to a laser. Macrophage cells keep the skin "clear" of debris, and while the collagen is busy "clearing," the epidermis regenerates automatically, thereby allowing melanocytes to return and the scar to be restored to the natural skin color.

Prompted by her findings, Dr. Schreibner had the idea of stimulating the same natural process of scar pigmentation, by using the "minor trauma" induced by a "dry needle" (i.e. without implanting pigment) rather than by laser. The epidermis was thus stimulated to undertake its own repigmentation.

To stimulate natural recoloration in small areas of vitiligo

Small areas of vitiligo can also be treated in this way. MCA can be a way of dealing with small, stable patches or edges only (see earlier explanation), so that either natural repigmentation can take place or so that the line between the area of white and normal skin can at least be toned down.

To improve the appearance of wrinkles

We have observed, especially when applying lipliners, that these regenerative "microtraumas" of the skin improve the appearance of the wrinkles and lines that form around the lips in the majority of people as they get older. Whether pigment is implanted or not, the process produces some very satisfactory results. Many clients notice that their lipstick no longer runs into these lines to form tiny, thin, red streaks.

To conclude, we can only say that the chapter on "multitrepannic collagen actuation" is still being written. Hopefully, great strides will be made over the next few years. It is, however, already a fascinating field to those who practice permanent makeup. What could be more satisfying than to be able to stimulate *the body* to correct its own small imperfections *all by itself*.

[1]This term, derived from the Greek, means "to make several small drill or bore holes."

[2]Author of the book *The Essence of Beauty*, Los Angeles, 1994. However, we would like to thank Kristanne Matzek of the American Institute of Permanent Color Technology for supplying us with the information given in this chapter.

[3]Cf. Zwerling, Walker, Goldstein, *Micropigmentation, State of the Art*, USA, 1993, p. 175 ff.

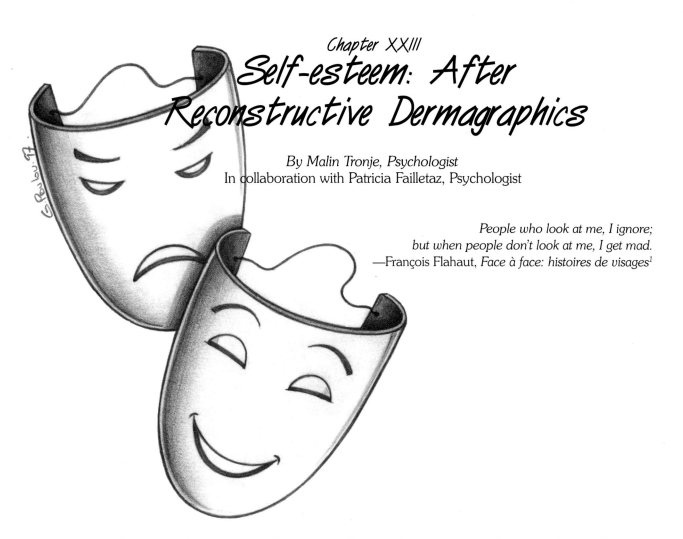

Chapter XXIII
Self-esteem: After Reconstructive Dermagraphics

By Malin Tronje, Psychologist
In collaboration with Patricia Failletaz, Psychologist

People who look at me, I ignore;
but when people don't look at me, I get mad.
—François Flahaut, *Face à face: histoires de visages*[1]

Our skin is always open to the scrutiny of others. It expresses, in a language that is silent and immediate, all that we do not say with words. A powerful means of identification and communication, the skin has always been an object that was looked after and often marked. The most ancient forms of marking are scarification and tattooing.

Historically, there are a number of reasons why people went in for tattooing. It could distinguish certain individuals within an ethnic group or it could indicate affiliation to a group or social class. Tattooing also figured in rituals to help an individual through a difficult period or to signify that he/she had reached an important stage in life. Cosmetics and makeup have their roots in the ancient custom of tribal markings.

But it was probably most frequently used as a means of seducing. We are all familiar with the frescos discovered in ancient Egyptian tombs that reveal how much the Egyptians prized their appearance and how important makeup was to them.

Apart from adorning the individual, makeup also creates a mask that acts as a screen between the individual and the people around him. With the help of makeup we can choose which aspect of our soul we wish to exhibit at any given moment. Makeup can therefore reveal what lies deepest within us or it can be a refuge from prying eyes.

Permanent makeup has been a part of our culture for several years now. It can be an alternative to traditional makeup or it can complement traditional makeup. A growing number of individuals have resorted to it for a variety of different reasons. It can be for the purpose of embellishment, as an affirmation of one's sensuality, to gain time, or to disguise a disfigurement resulting from an illness or accident. But whatever the motive, two reasons seem to crop up time and again: the desire to please oneself and the pleasure of pleasing.

But from where does this desire to please spring? Why does it matter how others see us, and how does it influence the way we see ourselves?

The gaze as a mirror

The influence of the eyes or gaze of those around us begins in early infancy – before we are even born. During pregnancy the parents imagine their future child. Their expectations and dreams create an "imaginary baby" that will partly determine how they regard their "real baby" when it is born. These images will be reflected in the way the parents look after their child and communicate with it. These interactions will contribute to the image the child gradually builds up of itself and will probably influence future relationships. Some people can spend their whole lives attempting to shake off these parental projections as they search for their own identity.

Jacques-Marie Lacan[2] describes this act of self-recognition, which emerges in an infant around the age of six months, as the "mirror stage." According to him, a child can recognize his own image in the mirror. He first perceives it as a real being, other than himself. Once he is able to understand that it is a reflected image he then begins to grasp the idea that it is his own image. The mirror allows him to see what he is and what he will become, and it is through the mirror that the infant forms his first notion of the "I."

The mother's gaze, and then that of others, will later replace the mirror, thus giving the child an identity. It could be said that the child becomes aware of himself through the awareness of others.

As adults, we play this same "mirror game." Our self-image is, in a way, dependent on the gaze of others. It would seem that the gaze of the "other" is always upon us; whether it is the mother's in early infancy, our peers in adolescence, indeed our social or professional groups as adults. Like the mirror, it influences our sense of belonging and the way we see ourselves.

All the time that body and mind are in complete harmony, this poses no problem. But what happens when our self-image, as reflected in others' eyes, does not correspond to what we are or to what we would like to be? How is it possible to live with a physical complex if the attitude of those around us is a constant reminder and confirmation of the fact? How does it feel to be full of life and energy when every time you look at your skin you are reminded of the passing of the years? One solution of course is to accept these as facts of life and learn to love ourselves as we are. But not all of us are strong enough to take responsibility for our own individuality, and it is sometimes difficult to be indifferent to mirrors and the gaze of others.

It is interesting how when inner and outer selves are in tune with one another we are barely conscious of our bodies. It is often the more unusual situations— stressful or emotional periods — that bring out these problems. And it is especially during or immediately after periods such as these that we decide it is time for a change and so begin to look into ways of making it happen.

Finding a new image

Most of us have, at one time or other, found ourselves wanting to change an aspect of our appearance following a pleasant or upsetting experience. It might mean a new outfit or a different hairstyle. It is almost as though we need to allow the emotionally charged event to physically manifest itself through a visible change in us. But what is it that makes us want to permanently change the appearance of our skin through cosmetic or reconstructive dermagraphics?

We all aspire to social integration and probably all want to be acknowledged and accepted for who and what we are. But it is not difficult to see how even mild physical disgust can shatter a person's confidence and turn one into a social recluse. In such a situation, a minor operation like permanent makeup can make a huge difference to the person who decides to go ahead with it. It could be the first step towards self-worth and a stepping stone leading to other projects. Whether visible or hidden by clothes, the end result can help a person change their attitude and at last begin to flourish. The people around will notice the change, confirm it in their eyes, and reinforce this new feeling of well being. In this way permanent makeup is once more linked with the ancient tradition of tattooing, marking an important transition in life.

However, it can happen that although the procedure is in every way a great success, the person might still not regain his or her self-confidence. It could be that the person's physical and psychological expectations were too high. If so, then the results can be such a terrible disappointment that, rather than relieving, they could re-open old wounds. Imagine a shy woman, lacking in self-confidence, who has a complex as a result of a facial blemish. Cosmetic surgery would not bring her out of herself unless she also changed her attitude to herself and the people around her. Moreover, any uncertainty on her part might be reinforced if, despite her new appearance, those around her continued to look at her in the same way. There is the added risk that, rather than deal with her deep-seated psychological problem, she will find some other imperfection that needs correcting in her quest for the impossible dream.

On the other hand, the same person can flourish if the results of the intervention correspond to her inner state. For she will want to proclaim her self-worth by showing a face or body that reflects her present state of mind. The intervention is then part of a process where the tattoo is the visible symbol of an inner transformation.

The problem might, at first glance, appear to be different when the person wants to hide the visual reminders of an accident or illness. For then it is more a question of regaining one's pre-accident or pre-illness image. In a situation like this, reconstructive dermagraphics is neither a return to the past nor the negation of a painful experience. Anyone choosing to opt for this kind of intervention must want to face their problem and allow someone from outside the medical profession to take care of their skin. The decision to do something about one's appearance can mark the end of a difficult period and give the individual the weapons he needs to defend himself and fight back. Inner and outer self, having been reconciled through the skin, mind, and body, can now walk side by side.

The art of getting into a client's skin

After a time, cosmetic procedures fade, but the effects last for years. It is therefore important that such procedures reflect the person's character, or at least those aspects the client wishes to reveal. Consequently, permanent makeup cannot, and must never be, a spur of the moment decision.

For optimum results it is important that the operation be carried out in an atmosphere of trust, by a technician who is not only technically competent but who has the necessary psychological and communication skills. It is absolutely essential for the technician to understand how the client sees herself and how she would *like* to see herself. Like the actor, the technician must get into their character's skin.

Honesty is also the best policy when it comes to dealing with clients. Together, practitioner and client must outline the strengths and weaknesses of the body, skin, and face. If the client is asking for the impossible from permanent makeup, the technician must help the client be more realistic and reach a happy compromise between dream and reality. To avoid disappointment or a nasty surprise, it is important that the client understands the procedure and the likely outcome. The technical and psychological aspects of a technician's skills must come together as the art is practiced on this thin surface that is our skin — the interface between body and soul.

Conclusion

Cosmetic practices and notions of beauty change with time and affect the way we regard others and ourselves. Over the last few years an increasing number of people have resorted to permanent makeup. Whilst the reasons will vary depending on the individual, they are all associated with the harmonization of outer appearance and inner state of mind. Permanent makeup is not a pointless, narcissistic exercise to the person who chooses to go in for it. It is an affirmation of the self that gives us an increased sense of well being. The physical and psychological are inextricably linked. And whoever changes one, inevitably changes the other. It is up to us to decide where to begin. Yet whatever steps an individual decides to take, he or she will improve peer-group integration and become an asset when it comes to dealing with everyday life.

[1]Flahaut, F. (1989). *Face à face: histoires de visages*. Paris, Plon.
[2]Lacan, J. (1966). *Le Stade du miroir comme formateur de la fonction du Je*, Ecrits, Paris, Seuil.

A Physician's Perspective: Permanent Makeup in Conjunction With Plastic and Cosmetic Surgery

By Dr. Ingrid Arion, Paris, France

Plastic Surgery, Facial Cosmetic Surgery

The similarities between and complementary aspects of Eleonora Habnit's work and mine immediately led us to discuss our respective passions. Her passion being permanent makeup, and mine plastic and cosmetic surgery to the face. Or, to be more precise: the reshaping of the face through the treatment of wrinkles, the restructuring of the cheekbones, the re-contouring of the lips, the rejuvenating of the eyes, etc.

Cosmetic and plastic surgery on the one hand, and permanent makeup on the other, both respond, or attempt to respond, to problems frequently associated with the effects or prevention of aging skin.

When it comes to the face, the most frequent requests we get during a consultation are for more attractive, neater skin; for more clearly-defined, or better shaped lips; for fuller, more "raised" eyebrows; as well as the softening and even — why not — the eradication of wrinkles.

Therapeutic treatments can respond to many of these requests, but as we are about to see through a study of the two areas of the face, the advantages of combining several methods are considerable.

For the sake of convenience, picture the face divided into two areas:

✓ The *upper* area, above the horizontal line that passes through the nostrils
✓ The *lower* area, below this line

Upper area (top half of the face)

Modern advances in the areas of plastic and cosmetic surgery means that we are now able to treat aging skin on the forehead as well as the lines and small wrinkles that develop around the eyes (crows' feet).

A combination of wrinkle treatment products and a course of injections into the muscle lifts the eyebrows, thus making the eyes look younger. The wrinkles of the forehead and around the eyes disappear.

Here the application of permanent makeup can be most useful, for it can be applied to re-accent sparse eyebrows, thereby livening up a listless-looking face

In my opinion it is essential that the cosmetic surgeon pass on to the permanent makeup technician information concerning any injections administered during an eyebrow lift operation. There is always a risk the eyebrow line might end up at the wrong height.

When a client wants almond-shaped eyes, she can of course opt for major cosmetic surgery: the "*mask lift*" (which entails raising the outside corner or external canthus of the eye). The application of eyeliner is a more minor operation that will create the desired effect but without trauma.

There is a great demand in both cosmetic and plastic surgery for the restructuring of the cheekbones. One answer, which has proven both satisfactory and long-term, is to combine re-modeling through a course of injections and a permanent makeup *blush* to accent the curve.

This symbiosis of cosmetic surgery and dermagraphics on the upper half of the face can also be implemented when it comes to improving the appearance of post-facelift scars. With time these can have a tendency to become more pronounced (white) as the pigmentation changes. Scars left by a cervico-facelift can be embarrassing as they are just in front of the ears. Permanent makeup is a clever way of disguising these types of problems.

Lower area (bottom half of the face)

Collaboration between doctor - cosmetic surgeon - permanent makeup technician, is, in my opinion, essential when it comes to beautifying and/or rejuvenating the lips. The effect on a client's general appearance of a combined lip contour (through permanent makeup) and lip reshape (by injecting into the lip vermilion) is quite spectacular. The mouth, if not the whole of the face, looks firmer and sharper.

This complementary benefit is actually even more important when the lips have undergone plastic or reconstructive surgery (to correct a cleft-lip or facial disfigurement following an accident).

Conclusion

The list is not exhaustive. The specialized areas we work in will continue to complement each other depending on the individual case and our professional judgment. To meet our patients' expectations, we who work in the field of plastic and cosmetic surgery increasingly must call upon the expertise of specialists in permanent makeup. To the great satisfaction of our clients, their art so often puts the finishing touches to our plastic and cosmetic surgery.

Chapter XXV

Herpes Labialis

When a client asks me for permanent makeup of the *lips*, the first question that springs to *my* lips is: do you get herpes labialis (more commonly known as cold sores or fever blisters)? Herpes labialis (its medical name is *herpes simplex* type 1, HVS1) is an extremely common and highly contagious virus, and its effects are as unpleasant as they are unattractive[1].

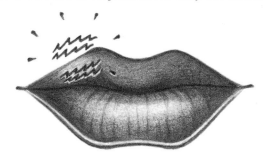

Around 90% of adults are carriers of herpes labialis, but only in a third of these does it manifest itself, either at regular or irregular intervals. It has a tendency to die down over the years but you will never be rid of it. If you have ever had a cold sore, even once, it is because you carry the virus

Under normal conditions (i.e. no eruption of blisters) the virus causing the attacks is dormant and might remain so for good. A sudden eruption could be due to a variety of factors: exposure to the sun, stress, fatigue, illness, menstruation, permanent makeup, etc. — not forgetting the impact our general health and state of mind might have. An outbreak can last anywhere from five to fifteen days.

Don't worry: herpes labialis does not mean you cannot go in for permanent makeup of the lips. However, to avoid adding futility to distress, here are four ways to counteract the virus.

Diet

Certain nutritional measures can give your immune system a natural boost: increase your lysine intake and decrease your arginine intake. Both are found in the foods we eat.

The best sources of lysine are: *fish, chicken, beef, milk, lamb, pork, beans, yeast, and soy.*

Arginine (which is to be avoided) is found in *hazelnuts, peanuts, walnuts, almonds, chocolate, sesame seeds, coconut, pistachio nuts, brown rice, and whole meal bread.*

American nutritionists recommend that, as a preventive measure, 500mg of lysine be taken a day and that during an attack, 1.5 to 3g be taken daily.

Homeopathy

Homeopathy is good when it comes to both prevention and cure.

At the onset of symptoms, take *one dose of Apis 9c.* An hour later (and then every two hours) take *3 granules of Rhus tox. 5c.*

Doses of *vaccinninum, 5-7-9-12 and 30c* taken at two weekly intervals (but four weeks between the penultimate and the last) are a useful measure against recurrent attacks. The treatment should be repeated once a year.

Creams, gels, ointments, and sticks

There are several products on the market (available over the counter) that deal with mild attacks. Examples are those containing the following ingredients: *acyclovir* (Zovirax™), *lyzozyme, tromandatine, zinc sulfate.*

In a fair number of cases, repeated applications at the onset of tingling will hopefully check the virus or at least accelerate the healing process.

Lyzozyme sticks can also be used to prevent an attack when you are suffering from an infectious disease or going through a stressful period. The same product, enriched with protection factor 12, is recommended for people who have a predisposition to solar herpes.

Tablets

If you are prone to severe attacks of herpes, a preventive measure like Zovirax™ tablets (active ingredient: *acyclovir*) taken three days before, the day of, and three days after treatment, is available only by prescription, as are Famvir™ (active ingredient: *famcyclovir*) and Valtrex™ (active ingredient: *valacyclovir*).

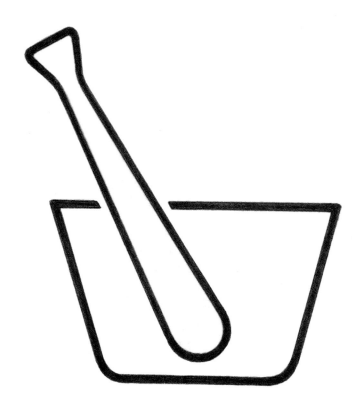

As you see, despite the fact that there is no effective vaccine or antiviral agent that can oust this undesirable guest from our system, there are fortunately several ways of dealing with herpes labialis.

[1]Some of the information in this chapter is from *Info-Santé-Service.*

Chapter XXVI
Permanent Makeup and MRIs

(Magnetic Resonance Imaging)

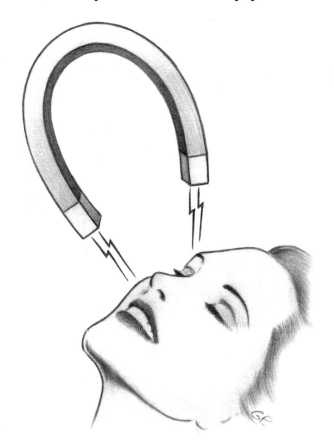

What does an MRI have to do with permanent makeup procedure?

Some radiologists, when performing MRI scans (not to be confused with X-rays), observed that patients who had permanent makeup/tattoos (especially on the eyelids) sometimes experienced a tingling sensation. They also found, to their surprise, that while the MRI had no adverse effect on the health of these patients, the images obtained were distorted.

These observations naturally led them to take a closer look at this phenomenon and undertake an in-depth study.

It would appear from studies so far, that the great majority of people who have undergone permanent makeup/tattooing experienced nothing in particular during an MRI, but that a small number of them experienced symptoms such as tingling or a slight burning sensation. In none of the cases studied was it necessary to stop the imaging process.

Some patients reported that their permanent makeup faded after an MRI scan. But this only happened when permanent makeup had been recently applied (no more than a month before the MRI scan).

What was extraordinary however was that in around 50% of cases the pigmentation showed up on the images. And in over 80% of these cases, the colors used were those most likely to contain iron oxide-based pigments, i.e. black, brown or flesh tones.

149

We asked Dr Jean-Chrétien Oberson, a Swiss specialist in radiodiagnostics, to subject a client (who, a month earlier, had undergone a lipliner and permanent makeup to her eyelids) to an MRI scan. The doctor did indeed see *"signs of minor distortions in the imaging, particularly of the eyes but less so of the lips."* In his opinion, this was due to *"the tattoo's fine metallic particles distorting the image,"* having become *"magnetized by the MRI scanner's powerful magnetic field."* Moreover, he pointed out that the patient had experienced *"mild stabbing pains in the eyelids the moment she came into contact with the machine's magnetic field."*

To conclude, we would like to stress that apart from the possibility of minor discomfort during a scan, permanent makeup/tattoo containing iron oxide-based pigments is not a health hazard. But anyone who knows they are about to undergo an MRI scan should inform the diagnostic technician or radiologist about their permanent makeup. As a result, even though the presence of this substance does not have a detrimental affect on an MRI, the radiologist will:

✓ See the distortion of the image, which would come as no surprise

✓ Prepare the patient for the possibility that she might feel some slight and temporary discomfort, particularly if the makeup was fairly recently applied.

However, be prepared, the MRI scanner will not be alone in reacting to the magnetic charm of your permanent makeup.

Chapter XXVII
Laser Tattoo Removal

What happens when that "little tattoo" becomes a "big taboo?"

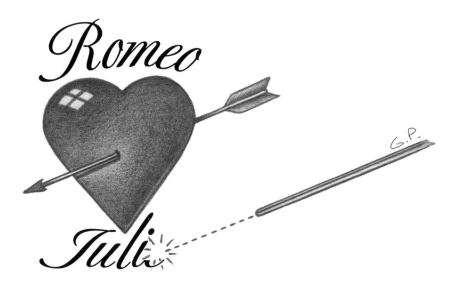

Removing tattoos is considered a *surgical operation* that neither permanent makeup technicians nor tattoo artists are prepared or authorized to do. They can, however:

- ✓ Cover the old design with a new one
- ✓ Go over it with flesh-colored pigment (not always attractive)

The advent of *"Q-Switched"* lasers, at the beginning of the 1990s, has revolutionized tattoo removal. They can remove pigments without leaving scars[1].

How do they work?

The principle upon which they work is that, for a fraction of a second, they emit (*"pulse"*) a beam of light the wavelength of which will depend on the pigment color. This beam passes through the epidermis and strikes only the pigment molecule without damaging the neighboring cells. The energy from the laser creates a "mini-explosion" that causes these molecules to fragment into smaller particles. These are then "digested" by the macrophages (the clearing up cells), a process that takes around three to four weeks.

How many sessions does it take?

Two to ten sessions, depending on the color and composition of the pigment and on how deep it has been implanted. For optimum results, the sessions are staggered over a period of one to two months.

Does it hurt?

The treatment is not painless, but it is not so bad that it requires anesthetic. Some say it is very much like the pain experienced during the tattooing process while others compare it to an elastic band twanging against the skin (the noise is in fact very similar!).

What are the immediate effects?

The skin immediately turns white and opaque. It can remain like that for around an hour, sometimes longer. The surrounding area turns red (erythema) and swells (edema). Then, as with a tattoo, small scabs form. These will eventually drop off around ten days later. It is advisable not to expose the treated area to the sun for at least two months after the final session.

Are there any unpleasant side effects?

Slight depigmentation of the treated area may occur. This is due to the fact that the energy emitted by the laser also absorbs the natural pigmentation (melanin). Once the tattoo has disappeared, the melanin returns, slowly but not always completely.

As you can see, dermapigmentation will not vanish with a wave of the magic wand. You cannot compare lasers — even the *"Q-Switched"* type — to the handy eraser you use to get rid of an unwanted pencil mark. There is no room for second thoughts — either on the part of the artist or his client. Whilst great advances are being made in the area of tattoo removal by laser, it is still a long process that requires a lot of patience.

[1]The following information is courtesy of Dr Isabelle Catomi, Paris and of the following institutes: Laser Centrum, Eindhoven, Holland and Laserase, Cosmetisch Laser Centrum, Antwerp, Belgium.

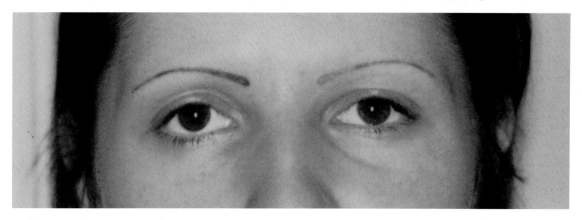

Eyebrows tattooed with black ink. Black ink should never be used in cosmetic tattooing. The color turns to blue-green.

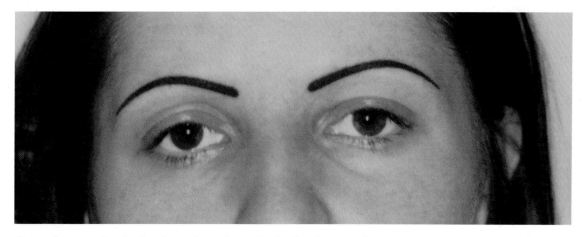

Camouflaging and reshaping the eyebrow. Immediately after the procedure.

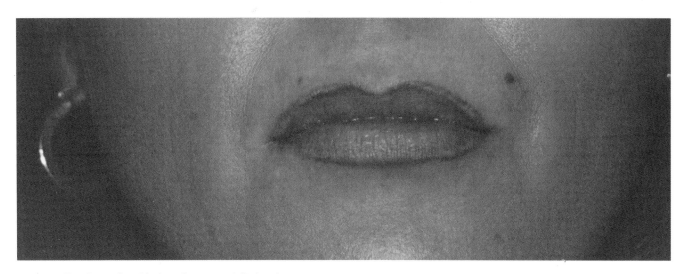

Poorly rendered lipliner by an unskilled technician.

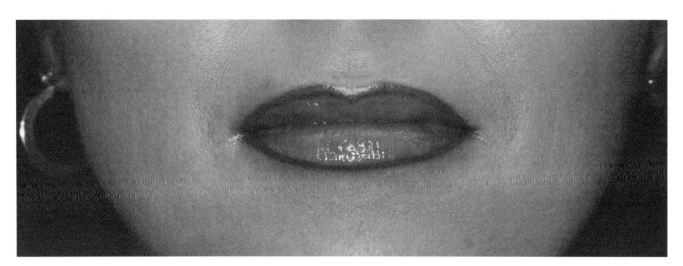

Camouflaging the dark lipliner. Immediately after the first procedure.

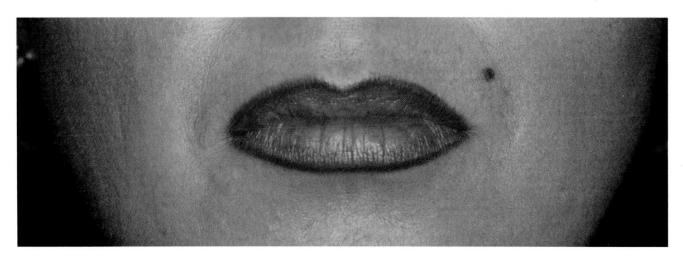

The final result after two procedures.

Chapter XXVIII
National Testing and Certification

By Dr. Kristanne Matzek[1], FAAM, Tustin, California

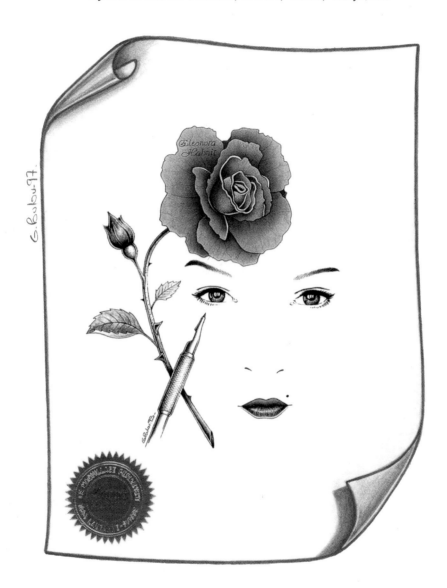

As permanent makeup becomes more popular, it is inevitable that regulatory agencies will begin to take a closer look at the technicians performing such procedures. If dermagraphics is to survive and become truly reputable in the eyes of the public and the medical specialties, we need to address the important issues of education, credentials, and ethics.

In 1994, a non-profit Academy was formed, with the sole purpose of "board certifying" technicians.

What is "Board Certification?"

A doctor practices medicine; an attorney practices law. Both lawyers and physicians are regulated by state agencies and associations, and must take exams before they are allowed to practice.

Cosmetologists, electrologists, aestheticians, and nurses are also regulated by state agencies and must take exams before they are allowed to work. Should the permanent makeup technician be any different?

How does a physician become board certified?

Most MD's go through four years of college, four years of medical school, a minimum one-year internship, and three years as a resident. Then they become board eligible to take the exam in their specialty. Are they still a doctor? Yes. Are they board certified? Not yet! In some cases, they take a written exam, get a score, and then advance to the oral portion of the exam at another date. Having a physician board certified, and having a regulatory agency, such as a board of medicine, protects the public. It tells a prospective patient that this physician has passed an exam to determine competency. It allows the public to have a place to voice a complaint, where action can be taken against a physician who wrongs that patient.

How do others become board certified?

When someone decides to become a cosmetologist, registered nurse, lawyer, doctor, etc., they go to a school approved by the board of education in their state. Once they graduate the training program, they apply to take their state board. Upon passing the boards, they become licensed or registered (such as licensed cosmetologists, registered nurses, registered electrologists, etc.) and, every year they pay an annual fee to that board to maintain their status and/or license. In many cases, continuing education units (CEU's) are required to keep the license current. If you decide to move to another state, you may have to take that state's board examination, unless there is a reciprocity agreement that grants you the right to work there without retaking an exam.

What about permanent makeup technicians?

Unfortunately, most states haven't established a separate board for permanent makeup technicians. Therefore, in most states, the Board of Health or Professional Licensing becomes responsible for regulating the technician, or at least for inspecting them if a complaint is made. In a sense, permanent makeup technicians are orphans! We don't have a state board that recognizes us or wants to regulate us. For electrologists, this scenario is not new. Not every state has a board of electrology, so many practitioners have relied on a national testing body to "certify" them. Our situation closely mirrors theirs.

The American Academy of Micropigmentation[2]

Since the individual states have not regulated technicians, we have to regulate ourselves. The American Academy of Micropigmentation (AAM) has established itself as a "testing body" created for the sole purpose of board certifying technicians. Using the American College of Surgeons board certification as a model, the AAM established itself in 1994 as a non-profit association and developed an examination to certify permanent makeup technicians. In 1998, the state of Maine adopted the criteria and made the exam mandatory for practicing technicians in their state.

As is the case for physicians in any specialty, taking the exam requires filling out and submitting an application. The technician must have been in practice for at least one year, then he or she becomes a "candidate" eligible to take the exam. The AAM exam consists of three parts: an oral exam, a written exam, and a practical exam.

Upon successful completion of the exam, a technician becomes "board certified," raising the level of credibility and professionalism he or she brings to the field. Further, the level of care in the application of permanent makeup is standardized, providing the patient with a win-win situation.

With permanent makeup becoming such a growing industry, the need for board certification is essential.

[1]www.aipct.com
[2]www.micropigmentation.org

Chapter XXIX
Permanent Makeup Associations

By Dr. Kristanne Matzek[1], FAAM, Tustin, California

The purpose of any permanent makeup association, indeed any professional association in general, is to educate its membership and publicize the benefits of treatment. Dues are paid to fund this campaign and contribute to the good of the industry.

This public relations program is designed for *all* technicians. In this way, all have equal opportunity to enjoy the publicity and share in its deductible expense. The more members the associations enroll, the less expensive but more effective the program becomes per member. These associations, through their editorials, newsletters, etc., educate the public on what to expect from proper treatment. The membership has to perform in accordance with a knowledgeable public. Incompetent and mediocre technicians will be forced to improve their skills or leave the profession altogether.

Why enroll?

The medical and dental professions spend millions of dollars each year to maintain their professional image. The associations expect to improve the status of the permanent makeup profession with the same techniques these professions use, only at a much more modest cost.

The final result of this enrollment will be a better-educated technician and a better-informed public. Both school enrollments and technicians' practices will proportionately increase. Unified licensing standards as well as recognition of permanent makeup as a dignified para-medical profession will result.

The American Academy of Micropigmentation[2]

Begun in 1994, this non-profit association offers board certification for permanent makeup technicians. An annual trade show in October brings technicians from around the world, seeking information, recognition, and credibility as practitioners.

Society of Permanent Cosmetic Professionals[3]

Started in 1991, this is a non-profit association that has dedicated itself to improving the training of technicians in the field.

Mandatory signing of a code of ethics brings a level of professionalism to this membership. Their annual trade show takes place in March, at different locations around the country — selected by the membership each year.

Annual dues provide a quarterly newsletter and recognition in the field.

[1]www.aipct.com
[2]www.micropigmentation.org
[3]www.spcp.org

Chapter XXX
State Laws and Regulations

*By Philippe Nordmann, Attorney at Law, LIC, OEC, HSG, Lausanne, Switzerland,
and Charles Zwerling[1], MD, FACS, FICS, Goldsboro, North Carolina*

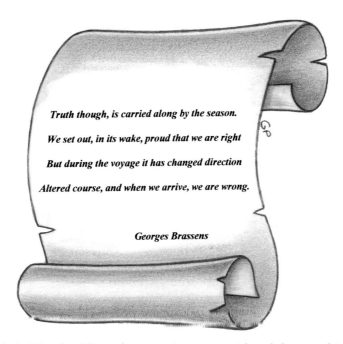

Truth though, is carried along by the season.

We set out, in its wake, proud that we are right

But during the voyage it has changed direction

Altered course, and when we arrive, we are wrong.

Georges Brassens

Tattooing was forbidden by Moses because it was considered the worship of idols. The Mosaic Law does seem to have been obeyed by most of his followers throughout the centuries. However, despite biblical injunctions, despite Muhammed I's prohibitions, despite decrees by the Roman Emperor Constantine, and despite more laws against or limiting tattoos for reasons of public health throughout the centuries, tattooing persists today. Indeed, the number of tattoo artists, professional and amateur, as well as the number of physicians and veterinarians who are doing tattooing for cosmetic purposes, is increasing at a phenomenal rate. Membership in regional, national, and international tattoo clubs is also increasing yearly.

With the advent of cosmetologists, aestheticians, manicurists, electrologists, and nurses performing dermagraphics, a number of the various state boards of medicine, nursing and/or cosmetology have had to address this issue. The various boards and agencies have struggled to deal with this rapidly growing field, and differ from state to state as to whether permanent makeup is deemed within their scope. The reader is urged to check with each state for precise clarification.

Of paramount concern, is protecting the public. How does the state go about this?

a) State licenses and investigations

When the state decides intervention is necessary, this can be done in one of two ways. The first is a *precautionary measure*, and involves subjecting the profession to a *license to practice* (e.g. doctors, lawyers, café-restaurants), a license that can be revoked in the event of malpractice. The second is *a posteriori*, and involves issuing an *investigation* order, which, for practical reasons, can only be done if an official complaint has been lodged. The law must make provision for the investigation, which cannot be effective unless it is accompanied by a range of sanctions in the case of particular professional regulations having been violated. These must also have been provided for under the law.

When it comes to permanent makeup, its pedigree was only established a few years ago, and the state (as we know) is a cumbersome machine, whose legislative wheels sometimes take years to start turning. However, we are hopeful that the recent extraordinary growth in the popularity of tattooing and permanent makeup will urge the authorities to grant these and other professions that involve "operating" on the human body (*body piercing*, etc.) official status.

b) State recognition of professional qualifications

There is, however, another way in which the state can guarantee a certain degree of public protection: the regulation of *professional qualifications,* through the setting up of recognized training courses and the issuing of state diplomas. Professionals who have not followed an appropriate course and who do not hold an official diploma, will then — at least if the state so wishes — be less "competitive" in the eyes of the public. The state will also have indirectly created an incentive for people who want to work in that particular field to get the proper training.

If the authorities were to take certain measures, the number of official training courses would increase. After all it is not unreasonable to expect that anyone entering a profession should have obtained a diploma. If no diploma exists, then the state will have to take responsibility for setting up official examinations — but not without first informing potential candidates how they should prepare for them. This comes back to advocating training courses, which, though neither guaranteed nor required by the state, are however – euphemistically – strongly supported by it, enough de facto to acquire official status.

c) Professional associations

For want of state recognition, networks set up by the various professional associations have a crucial role to play. They disseminate information, provide courses for in-service training, and publish journals that prove invaluable to any isolated professional who, without them, would find it difficult to keep abreast of developments. The absence of official state control does, in a way, prejudice the nature and efficiency of such associations. However, their genuineness will eventually gain them official state recognition.

State laws and/regulations

1) Prohibition of the tattooing of minors
This is one of the only common features among the fifty states. A minor is designated as a person under the age of 18; in Texas, however, it is unlawful to tattoo any persons under the age of 21. Some cities and counties have local ordinances that restrict or regulate tattooing, including the allowance of parental consent for minors.

2) States regulating permanent makeup
Because facial dermagraphics is considered tattooing, many states have placed permanent makeup alongside body piercing and tattooing in the regulatory pool. Currently, most states have licensing requirements.

Some legal considerations...

How does the technician protect herself? Between the client who is asking for a permanent makeup/tattoo and the professional provider there is a contractual agreement. This is significant because all dermagraphics in a way constitutes an assault — albeit voluntary — on physical integrity. But we should not confuse such an assault with an unlawful act, such as injury inflicted during an act of aggression. The "physical assault" resulting from permanent makeup/tattoo can be likened to that occasioned during medical or dental treatment.

a) The importance of "informed consent"
The client must have been supplied with the full facts concerning the treatment he/she will undergo. Consent should only be given once the client is in full possession of the facts.

Practitioners should not limit themselves to replying to questions raised by the client, for the latter may *not know* that a particular question needs to be raised. It is therefore up to professionals to *anticipate* the questions, which, thanks to their experience, they will be well-placed to answer. They must inform the client that the makeup is permanent (and not simply "semi-permanent") and they must also point out that, in some instances, the makeup can fade fairly rapidly. They must draw the client's attention to certain risks (allergies, herpes). They must also endeavor to obtain as much information as possible regarding the client's medical history and present state of health. In short, they will place the ball firmly in the client's court (and at the same time in their own!). Ideally, they should devise written questionnaires and draw up lists of all the points that must be covered: after all, no pilot would dream of taking off until he had been through the items on his *checklist*.

b) *Responsibility of means/results*

In medicine, it is generally admitted that although a practitioner cannot guarantee to cure a patient, he is duty bound to do *everything within his power* and *according to the rulebook* to achieve this. The same principles apply to dermagraphics. Professionals are expected to:

- use approved techniques
- maintain standards of hygiene and use sterilized equipment
- keep abreast of recent developments, at home and abroad

The distinction between "means" and "results" is of paramount importance when it comes to determining whether or not, from an aesthetic point of view, a result is satisfactory. Of course, as we have already said, taste is relative. But we must be able to judge if the work has been carried out according to the rulebook or if the practitioner has been negligent.

As far as unpleasant side effects are concerned (allergies, infections), the practitioner will be questioned in order to ascertain whether all necessary precautionary measures (as laid down by the profession) were taken. The practitioner will also be asked whether the client's "informed consent" was obtained, i.e. whether the possibility of such side effects was pointed out. Slight though the risks are, they cannot not be entirely ruled out.

It is sometimes difficult to judge the results when it comes to reconstructive applications (from the point of view of results as opposed to means). It would not be realistic to demand a "perfect result" from practitioners as they are working on damaged skin.

We shall begin with the premise that the expectations of *the patient* are less precise than those of a candidate for permanent makeup. The former *knows what he/she no longer wishes to see* (his/her present condition) but has no idea what the final result should be, except that it should be better than it is at present.

Practitioners are therefore less "guided" by their clients than they would be when applying permanent makeup. Moreover, they are dangerously "free" when it comes to deciding what kind of operation to carry out and how to conduct it. Consequently, they will have to give their clients a much more detailed description of what they will be doing. The client will be more informed in his/her consent than with permanent makeup.

The freedom of practitioners is a great responsibility. They hold in their hands the future confidence and hope of that patient. If they have any doubts whatever, they will have to withdraw so as to avoid aggravating the condition. A photograph should always be taken of the original condition. This is virtually obligatory when it comes to reconstructive applications so that when the treatment is finished no blame can be attached to the practitioner — another reason why it is essential to act from within professional associations, to create them as the need arises, and, until something better comes along, to ask clients (so that their rights are safeguarded) to send for detailed information on treatments and qualified practitioners. The practitioner's experience and high professional standards are, when all is said and done, the best guarantee a client can have.

[1]www.micropigmentation.org

Conclusion

"What are generally regarded as purely feminine tastes: the pursuit of comfort and convenience, the love of adornment and entertainment, curiosity, etc. [...] are aspects of civilization. [...] Progress is not controlled by sober, rigid virtues but by vain, hedonistic proclivities and curiosity. The former is quite content with a simple life. The Spartans invented nothing but a few gloomy aphorisms. We can safely say that in any society, the more women are subjugated, the crueler that same society is. Throughout history the negation of feminine influence has always been a sign of social regression...[1]"

So aptly put — need one say more?

Permanent makeup is indeed an aspect of civilization and not just a passing fad, a "flash in the pan." Today it is coveted by all who love to show themselves to advantage, in other words...all of us! Far from being synonymous with routine, it is a base upon which we may still run riot with a pencil.

And, as a final touch, adding a delightful twist to our wicked pleasure, we might well be dressed and ready to go out, but now we are the ones who are kept waiting...

I don't understand how a woman
can go out looking a mess:
for it could be the day she has a date with destiny...
—Gabrielle (Coco) Chanel

[1]Mosca and Bouthoul, *Histoire des doctrines politiques*, Petite Bibliothèque Payot, Paris 1966, p. 341.